SCHIZOPHRENIA

SCHIZOPHRENIA
Recent Biosocial Developments

Edited by

Costas N. Stefanis, M.D.

and

Andreas D. Rabavilas, M.D.

Department of Psychiatry
Eginition Hospital
Athens, Greece

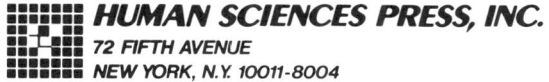 **HUMAN SCIENCES PRESS, INC.**
72 FIFTH AVENUE
NEW YORK, N.Y. 10011-8004

Printed in the United States of America
987654321

Library of Congress Cataloging-in-Publication Data

Schizophrenia : recent biosocial developments.

  1. Schizophrenia—Physiological aspects.
2. Schizophrenia—Social aspects.   I. Stefanis,
C. N. (Costas N.)   [DNLM: 1. Schizophrenia.
WM 203 S33797]
RC514.S3363   1987   616.89′82   86-27353
ISBN 0-89885-345-1

CONTENTS

CONTRIBUTORS

Yrjö O. Alanen, M.D. Department of Psychiatry, University of Turku, Finland.

Costas G. Alexopoulos, M.D. Department of Internal Medicine, Evangelismos Hospital, Athens, Greece.

Joanne D. Bergiannaki, M.D. Department of Psychiatry, Athens University Medical School, Eginition Hospital, Athens, Greece.

Joseph E. Comaty, M.S. Illinois State Psychiatric Institute, Chicago, Illinois.

Timothy J. Crow, M.D. Division of Psychiatry, Clinical Research Centre, Northwick Park Hospital, Harrow, England.

John M. Davis, M.D. Illinois State Psychiatric Institute, Chicago, Illinois.

Robert Giel, M.D. World Health Organization Collaborating Center, Department of Social Psychiatry, Groningen, Netherlands.

George Gournas, M.D. Department of Psychiatry, Community Mental Health Center, Athens University Medical School, Eginition Hospital, Athens, Greece.

Heinz Häfner, M.D., Ph.D. Central Institute of Mental Health, Mannheim, Federal Republic of Germany.

John Hatzimanolis, M.D. Department of Psychiatry, Athens University Medical School, Eginition Hospital, Athens, Greece.

Wolfram an der Heiden, M.S. Central Institute of Mental Health, Mannheim, FRG.

9

Philip G. Janicak, M.D. Illinois State Psychiatric Institute, Chicago, Illinois.

Anne Kaljonen, M.D. Department of Psychiatry, University of Turku, Finland.

Aphrodite Kapsali, M.D. Department of Psychiatry, Community Mental Health Center, Athens University Medical School, Eginition Hospital, Athens, Greece.

John Kibouris, M.D. Department of Psychiatry, Athens University Medical School, Eginition Hospital, Athens, Greece.

Vassilis Kontaxakis, M.D. Department of Psychiatry, Athens University Medical School, Eginition Hospital, Athens, Greece.

Juhani Laakso, M.D. Department of Psychiatry, University of Turku, Finland.

Aris Liakos, M.D. Department of Psychiatry, Ioannina University Medical School, Ioannina, Greece.

John A. Liappas, M.D. Psychophysiological Laboratory, Athens University Medical School, Department of Psychiatry, Eginition Hospital, Athens.

Sotiris Loukas, Ph.D. Department of Psychiatry, Ioannina University Medical School, Ioannina, Greece.

Sineke ten Horn, Ph.D. World Health Organization Collaborating Center, Department of Social Psychiatry, Groningen, Netherlands.

Urania Machera, M.D. Department of Psychiatry, Athens University Medical School, Eginition Hospital, Athens, Greece.

Michael Madianos, M.D. Department of Psychiatry, Community Mental Health Center, Athens University Medical School, Eginition Hospital, Athens, Greece.

Manolis Markianos, Ph.D. Department of Psychiatry, Athens University Medical School, Eginition Hospital, Athens, Greece.

Marios Markidis, M.D. Department of Psychiatry, Athens University Medical School, Eginition Hospital, Athens, Greece.

Sarnoff A. Mednick, Ph.D., M.D. Department of Psychiatry, Psykologisk Institute, Kommunehospitalet, Copenhagen, Denmark.

Yiannis G. Papakostas, M.D. Department of Psychiatry, Athens University Medical School, Eginition Hospital, Athens, Greece.

Josef Parnas, M.D. Department of Psychiatry, Psykologisk Institute, Kommunehospitalet, Copenhagen, Denmark.

Carlo Perris, M.D. Umea University, Department of Psychiatry III & WHO Collaborating Centre for Research and Training in Mental Health, Umea, Sweden.

Andreas D. Rabavilas, M.D. Psychophysiological Laboratory, Athens University Medical School, Department of Psychiatry, Eginition Hospital, Athens, Greece.

Viljo Räkkölainen, M.D. Department of Psychiatry, University of Turku, Finland.

Riitta Rasimus, M.D. Department of Psychiatry, University of Turku, Finland.

Pantelis Rinieris, M.D. Department of Psychiatry, Athens University Medical School, Eginition Hospital, Athens, Greece.

Paul N. Sakkas, M.D. Department of Psychiatry, Athens University Medical School, Eginition Hospital, Athens, Greece.

Georgia Sakellariou, M.D. Department of Psychiatry, Athens University Medical School, Eginition Hospital, Athens, Greece.

Norman Sartorius, M.D. World Health Organization, Geneva, Switzerland.

Fini Schulsinger, M.D. Department of Psychiatry, Psykologisk Institute, Kommunehospitalet, Copenhagen, Denmark.

Hanne Schulsinger, Ph.D. Department of Psychiatry, Psykologisk Institute, Kommunehospitalet, Copenhagen, Denmark.

Contantin R. Soldatos, M.D. Department of Psychiatry, Athens University Medical School, Eginition Hospital, Athens, Greece.

Costas N. Stefanis, M.D. Department of Psychiatry, Athens University Medical School, Eginition Hospital, Athens, Greece.

Timothy W. Teasdale, Ph.D. Division of Psychiatry, Clinical Research Center, Nocthwick Park Hospital, Harrow, England.

Stavroula Theodoropoulou-Vaidaki, M.D. Second Psychiatric Unit, Dromokaition Hospital, Athens, Greece.

George Tolis, M.D. Department of Psychiatry, Athens University Medical School, Eginition Hospital, Athens, Greece.

Vlassis Tomaras, M.D. Department of Psychiatry, Community Mental Health Center, Athens University Medical School, Eginition Hospital, Athens, Greece.

Eugenio Torre, M.D. Department of Mental Hygiene, University of Pavia, Pavia, Italy.

Gregory Vaslamatzis, M.D. Department of Psychiatry, Athens University Medical School, Eginition Hospital, Athens, Greece.

John K. Wing, M.D., Ph.D. MRC Social Psychiatry Unit, Institute of Psychiatry, London.

Stavroula Yannitsi, M.D. Department of Psychiatry, Ioannina University Medical School, Ioannina, Greece.

INTRODUCTION

C.N. Stefanis

According to rough estimates, over 20 million people in the world suffer from what is known today as schizophrenia. Afflicting mostly the young, and resulting in most cases in lifelong distress and impaired functioning, it imposes a heavy emotional and financial burden on its victims' families, and entails an immeasurable societal cost in terms of loss of productivity and provision of care. In short, it constitutes a major public health problem that cuts across all racial, cultural, and sociopolitical barriers.

Its diachronic nature is evidenced by abundant descriptions in the ancient literature of individuals with behavioral manifestations that are currently used as diagnostic criteria for schizophrenia. Concepts and attitudes towards this condition varied in time and differed from culture to culture; but its basic features were invariably recognized as indicating a substantial deviance from the norm. It became an issue of medical concern only about 150 ago, when it was described as an illness and emerged as the core subject of the science and practice of psychiatry. In fact, the birth of psychiatry as a medical specialty is closely associated with schizophrenia. It is mainly schizophrenia that enabled psychiatry to acquire its own professional autonomy from neurology and applied psychology. The development of the theory and practice of psychiatry has in many respects been determined by its efforts to diagnose schizophrenia reliably, to formulate plausible explanations of its symptoms, to understand its nature, and to discover effective means for its treatment.

The detailed description of a case and the introduction of the term *demence precose* by Morel in 1860; the systematic study of a large number of cases and their nosological categorization by Kraepelin at the turn of the century; the syndromal approach by Bleuler, who also coined the term "schizophrenia" in 1911; the formulation of diagnostic criteria by Schneider in the thirties; the impregnation of clinical thinking by the psychodynamic theory in the postwar years; the advent of neuroleptic chemotherapy in the early fifties, and finally, the recent upsurge of the deinstitutionalization and community care movement, are not merely all successive developmental stages in the medical history of schizophrenia, but also landmarks in the evolutionary course of psychiatry as a medical discipline, and healing profession.

Ever since its "medicalization," schizophrenia has become the target of vigorous research and the ground on which validity of hypotheses advanced by the various schools of thought in psychiatry has been tested. In the past 30 years in particular, research in various aspects of schizophrenia has burgeoned, and a wealth of data has been accumulated, yet a global understanding of the condition is lacking and its nature still remains an elusive puzzle. Even the validity of its own diagnosis is disputed. Long and strenuous efforts to corroborate clinical judgment by externally valid criteria have failed. We still depend for diagnosis entirely on clinical symptoms, none of which is stable in time or pathognomonic for the illness. Delineation from other psychiatric disorders in a great percentage of cases still depends on long-term observation and disputable treatment response trials.

Moreover, despite advances in elucidating biological and psychological mechanisms underlying its clinical manifestations, the etiology of the illness has not been clarified. Advances in treatment enabled psychiatrists and allied professionals to improve substantially the quality of life of patients with schizophrenic disorders, to relieve them from their symptoms and reduce their disabilities. However, expectations for a radical cure have not, as yet, been fulfilled and no imminent breakthroughs in this field are in sight. Schizophrenia still remains a challenge for psychiatrists and behavioral scientists alike. The task to unravel its enigmatic nature and master it by curative means is daunting. Nevertheless, substantive progress has already been made, and part of this is portrayed in this volume.

The Department of Psychiatry of Athens University was privileged to sponsor a symposium, held in Athens in October 1984, "Schizophrenia: Recent Biosocial Developments."

In this meeting, invited speakers of worldwide reputation for their expertise in specific areas of current research in schizophrenia, and staff members of the hosting department involved in ongoing related studies were given the opportunity to exchange views, to report original findings from their work, and to present a comprehensive and up-to-date account of current trends and future perspectives in both basic research and management strategies of schizophrenic disorders.

Out of the many papers presented in the meeting, those that dealt with issues in the forefront of research interest and those that qualified for incorporation into a unified body of knowledge, suited for the needs of this volume, were selected. Still, there is a great variability among the papers in their thematic orientation, length, and style. This could hardly be avoided, inasmuch as the intention was neither to compile a textbook on schozphrenia nor to limit the scope of the volume by restricting its content to a highly specific area of scientific and professional concern.

By grouping the selected papers together according to their primary area of interest and ordering them sequentially, four distinct, but interconnected, thematic entities emerged: etiology and pathogenetic mechanisms; psychopathology; treatment; and finally, management of schizophrenia in the frame of mental health services and complementary care systems.

The first contribution is a most informative and authoritative survey of WHO's international programs for schizophrenia, by N. Sartorius, the head of WHO's division of mental health. This survey, in addition to providing valuable information on methods developed and results obtained in international collaborative studies, sweeps through practically all issues that are further elaborated by the subsequent papers, and serves as a sort of introduction to the whole volume.

In the field of etiology of schizophrenia, there are four contributions. The first deals with the central issue of the role of genetic and environmental factors in the causation of schizophrenic disorders. This is dealt with by Schulsinger *et al.*, of Copenhagen in their paper, which is based on a large body of data accumulated throughout the years in the framework of the worldwide known longitudinal prospective study of high-risk groups in Denmark. The possible contribution of viral infections in the etiology of schizophrenia, an issue vigorously discussed in recent literature, is thoroughly reviewed by a pioneer investigator in this field, Dr. T. Crow *et al.*, of England. Adjacent to Dr. Crow's views are the original research findings by S. Theodoropoulou *et al.* of Athens in their paper on the immunological state of schizophrenic patients. The issue of possible hypersensitivity of the brain's dopaminergic system as a biochemical factor contributing to the etiology of schizophrenia has been approached by Hatzimanolis *et al.* of Athens by a neuroendocrine controlled investigation of nonmedicated schizophrenics.

In the field of psychopathology there are also four contributions. The first is by C. Perris from Umea, Sweden. Perris, who has gained an international reputation by his substantial contribution to clarifying diagnostic issues in psychiatry, presents an extensive and thorough study on the relation of cycloid psychosis to schizophrenia. Markidis *et al.* from Athens applied a linguistic methodology, tinted with philosophical thinking, in their attempt to approach the problem of speech disturbance in patients with schizophrenia. On the other hand, Liakos and his group from Ioanina, Greece, provide evidence, based on their own elaborately designed studies, of the effect of treatment, psychopathology, arousal, and anxiety on the cognitive performance of schizophrenics. Finally, Rabavilas *et al.* of Athens present additional data from their long-range study on brain laterality and psychopathology in order to support the view of a left hemispheric activation in patients with paranoid schizophrenia.

In the field of treatment there are also four contributions. The two papers, one by Alanen *et al.* from Turku, Finland, and the other by Davis *et al.* of Chicago are outstanding contributions. Alanen and his group present at length a detailed account of their results obtained by the application of a global psychotherapeutic approach to schizophrenic disorders. Davis and his group, on the other hand, in a display of high-quality authorship, manage to condense their extensive knowledge of the pharmacotherapy of schizophrenia in a most informative and amply documented text. A notable addition to the existing literature on the role of opiate peptides in schizophrenia derives from the short paper of Papakostas of Athens, who reports essentially negative results by naloxone treatment of schizophrenic patients with hallucinations. The ECT treatment of schizophrenia remains a controversial issue. Nevertheless, there is still room for further research. Soldatos *et al.* of Athens present preliminary results of their study indicating that nocturnal prolactin secretion in response to ECT may serve as an early prognostic index of ECT's efficacy in patients with schizophrenic disorders.

Last, in the field of management of schizophrenia in the frame of mental health services, there are six papers. They are all original contributions in an area of growing concern for mental health professionals, policy makers, and the public at large. The introductory paper is by Hafner and Heiden from the Central Institute of Mental Health in Mannheim, FRG. It brings forth and pragmatically deals with a wide range of issues associated with the social aspects of schizophrenia and the organization, effectiveness, and cost of mental health services. Based on a highly sophisticated evaluation of services in their own institute, and on comparative figures from elsewhere, the authors provide a comprehensive and documented appraisal of the newly emerging mental health care systems. In a similarly documented presentation, C. Perris of Umea furnishes his own firsthand experience from the implementation of a decentralized, sectorized, and community-based care system in a northern county of Sweden.

Coping with Schizophrenia at Home is the title of the paper by which J. Wing from London offers his own substantial contribution to this volume. In dealing with this crucial issue, Dr. Wing manages in a masterly way to combine the disciplinary rules of the social sciences with the emotional approach of the psychiatrist, and to bring us as close as we can get to patients' personal and family lives. In the next paper, Madianos *et al.* of Athens present their stimulating findings from a prospective, longitudinal study on the effect of family atmosphere on the course of chronic schizophrenia. Finally, two very timely papers provide a documented, rather than impressionistic, evaluation of the reform in mental health services in Italy. The widely discussed "Italian experiment" that aroused worldwide attention and still remains a controversial issue among professionals and the public alike, is viewed separately by an Italian and a Netherlander.

E. Torre from Pavia, in his chapter, "Deinstitutionalization: Alternatives to Mental Hospitals in Italy," outlines the historical background of the conception and implementation of the Italian Mental Health Act and attempts to evaluate critically its effectiveness by presenting findings from his own studies. The fundamental contribution of these findings is that figures and hard data are also being recognized as important in supporting ideological aspirations. R. Giel, a well-known social psychiatrist from Groningen, offers his own assessment of the Italian Act by comparing it with the mental health care system in Holland. His own firsthand observations are further supported in his paper by the comparative results obtained by two cohorts of patients, one in Trieste and the other in Chronigen, in the framework of the WHO study of mental health services in pilot study areas in Europe.

As we have already mentioned, schizophrenia, or the group of schizophrenias, as Bleuler first pointed out, most likely is not an homogeneous illness entity. Despite progress, neither has its enigmatic nature been revealed nor is a drastic cure for all its symptoms and disabilities currently available. Information derived from the biological, psychological, epidemiological, and social investigations remains fragmentary and cannot be integrated into a holistic model and lead to a unified concept of what is currently diagnosed as schizophrenia. The current state of fragmented knowledge is reflected in the contents of this volume. Nevertheless, it is only through the process of amassing seemingly disparate empirical data that we can attain the critical body of knowledge that will allow a concept of schizophrenia as a meaningful "whole" to emerge.

It is the editor's hope that this volume will contribute to this end.

I wish to express my deep appreciation to all the authors for their valuable contributions. I wish also to express my warm thanks to my secretary, Ms. Amalia Vlachodimitropoulou, for her competent and devoted assitance.

Athens, November 8, 1986

Part I

GENETIC, BIOCHEMICAL, AND IMMUNOLOGICAL FACTORS

Chapter 1

SOLVING THE CONUNDRUM OF SCHIZOPHRENIA

Who's Contribution

Norman Sartorius, M.D.

Some 20 million people in the world suffer from schizophrenia. The disease usually starts early and often has a chronic, disabling course. Treatment, unless rationalized, can be expensive, and the losses in terms of working capacity are staggering. Members of patients' family experience disadvantages because of the stigma attached to the diseased and his relatives. Schizophrenia is a major public health problem.

Though there have been advances in our knowledge about schizophrenia in the past few decades, nothing allows us to surmise that the causes of schizophrenia will soon become known, nor that the prevention of the disorder will become possible in the immediate future. The increasing complexity of human society and the disruption of social networks often accompanying economic growth raise the probability that schizophrenia will result in disability significantly larger than ever before.

Treatment of schizophrenia has been developed to a level at which it can be said that suffering of the patient can be reduced and his abnormal behavior controlled. The duration of the disorder, however, can be influenced much less readily and this fact coupled with the increase of the numbers of young adults—the population group at highest risk for schizophrenia—allows the prediction that the prevalence of schizophrenia will significantly grow over the next few decades.

These facts were among the reasons that made the World Health Organization pay special attention to the problem of schizophrenia and launch or stimulate studies aiming at a better understanding of schizophrenia and at finding ways to deal with it. These fall into three broad groups aiming at:

(a) an improved understanding of the nature of schizophrenia, and its form, course, and outcome in different sociocultural settings;

(b) an improvement of the methods of treatment of schizophrenia;

(c) learning about ways in which health and other social services can best apply knowledge about schizophrenia in the provision of care, in programs of rehabilitation, and in mental health education of the general population.

STUDIES OF THE FORM, COURSE, OUTCOME, AND FREQUENCY OF SCHIZOPHRENIA IN DIFFERENT CULTURES

The basis for work in this area was laid in the early 1960s following the recommendations of an expert committee on epidemiology of mental disorders (WHO 1960).[1] The committee urged that WHO should develop methods which will allow a standardization of assessment of psychiatric patients in different cultures; that it should carry out comparative studies of mental disorders seen in different cultures; and that it should promote the use of these methods in epidemiological studies and in the training of mental health workers.

Special attention was to be given to the standardization of psychiatric diagnosis, classification, and statistics. A 10-year program has been carried out in this area resulting in proposals for the international classification of mental and neurological diseases, in the development of glossaries of diagnostic terms, and in a number of publications. New methods of investigating the diagnostic process were developed and a network of individuals and institutions interested in this area and collaborating in WHO's program and among themselves.[2]

The first of a number of international meetings in this program, convened to debate the classification and explore issues of diagnosis was focused on schizophrenia.

A few years later, the first major WHO-coordinated study on schizophrenia was launched. It was seen as a pilot study (the International Pilot Study of Schizophrenia) preparing the ground for in-depth studies on schizophrenia and other mental disorders. The aim of this study was thus to tackle certain basic methodological problems and to answer questions about the nature and distribution of schizophrenia.

There were three major methodological questions:

1. Is it feasible to carry out a large-scale international psychiatric study requiring the coordination and collaboration of psychiatrists and mental health workers from different theoretical backgrounds and from widely separated countries with different cultures and socioeconomic conditions?

2. Is it possible to develop standardized research instruments and procedures for psychiatric assessment that can be reliably applied in a variety of cultural settings?

3. Can teams of research workers be trained to use such instruments and procedures so that comparable observations can be made both in developed and developing countries?

The major questions about the nature and distribution of schizophrenia that this study was intended to explore were:

1. In what sense can it be said that schizophrenic disorders exist in different parts of the world?

2. Are there groups of schizophrenic patients with similar characteristics present in every one of the countries studies?

3. Are there groups of schizophrenic patients whose symptoms differ in form or content from one country to another, and if so, are such differences the result of variations in diagnostic practice or are they true cultural differences in the manner of presentation of the various types of schizophrenia?

4. Does the clinical course and social outcome of schizophrenia in one country or group of countries differ from that in other countries?

5. How do the characteristics of schizophrenic patients compare with those of other psychoses in various countries?

6. Does the course of other psychoses differ from country to country?

In order to answer the questions outlined above, a comparative prospective study was designed. A series of psychotic patients was selected from among those contacting psychiatric services in nine countries. These patients were examined in a systematic and standardized fashion, and as many as possible have been followed up 2 and 5 years after the initial examination. The centers that participated in this study were Cali (Colombia), Taipei (China), Prague (Czechoslovakia), Aarhus (Denmark), Agra (India), Ibadan (Nigeria), Moscow (USSR), London (UK), and Washington (USA). Each field research center assessed all patients contacting it with two screens, a demographic screen and a psychosis screen. These screens were designed to select patients with functional psychoses who would be likely to be available for long-term follow-up.

The Psychosis Screen identified all of those patients who passed the Demographic Screen who did not meet any one of a number of exclusion criteria and who met at least one of a number of inclusion categories.

Exclusion criteria were chosen to screen out (a) chronic patients, and (b) patients whose conditions may have been caused or significantly influenced by an organic condition. Inclusion categories were symptoms rather than diagnostic labels. Inclusion categories were divided into (a) those whose presence automatically qualified the patient for inclusion, regardless of degree of symptomatology, and (b) those considered as a basis for inclusion only if present in severe degree. The first group consisted of delusions, hallucinations, gross psychomotor disorder, and definitely inappropriate and unusual behavior. The second group consisted of social withdrawal, disorders of form of thinking, overwhelming fear, disorders of affect, self-neglect, and depersonalization.

In all, the study population consisted of 1,202 patients, divided approximately equally over the nine centers. Of these patients 811 had a center diagnosis of schizophrenia, 164 of affective psychosis, 29 of paranoid psychosis, 73 of other psychoses, 71 of neurotic depression, and 54 had other diagnoses.

The design of the IPSS did not include a specific attempt to select series of patients who were representative samples of all schizophrenic patients or of all patients with other functional psychoses seen at the centers. Nevertheless it is obviously of interest to have some idea of the degree to which the IPSS patients are typical of all patients seen at the centers. The collaborating investigators were asked therefore to give their impressions about the typicality of the series of patients from their centers. It was the general impression that, taking into consideration that very young, very old, and chronic patients were excluded by design, the schizophrenic patients and the patients with affective psychoses included in the IPSS were for the most part typical, with regard to clinical characteristics, of all such relatively acute patients within the stated age-range admitted to the centers.

Each of the 1202 patients received an intensive initial evaluation by the research team at the field research center. Each evaluation took a total of about 5 hours and resulted in the accumulation of some 1600 items of information. This information was elicited through the use of a series of standardized instruments developed or adapted for the study. Eight such instruments were used in the study, of which the three basic ones were the Present State Examination (PSE), the Psychiatric History Schedule (PH) and the Social Description Schedule (SD). A full description of the instruments and reliability data about their use is presented in Volume 1, of the IPSS Report, (WHO, 1973).

The study provided positive answers to the methodological questions posed in the study: The investigation demonstrated that it is possible to carry out effectively a large-scale transcultural investigation of psychiatric disorders; that transculturally applicable· instruments for psychiatric research can be produced; and that teams of research workers can be trained to use standardized research instruments and procedures so that comparable observations can be made, both in developed and developing countries.

Questions about the nature and distribution of schizophrenia were approached by analysis of the psychopathology of patient groups, application of computer-simulated diagnosis, cluster analysis, and the identification and description of a concordant group of schizophrenia on which three methods of classification agree.

The results of analysis of the psychopathology of patient groups and the application of computer-simulated diagnosis indicated that the major functional psychoses are present in each of the centers' studies and that there were some groups of schizophrenic patients who had center-specific characteristics. A follow-up study has been carried out in all the centers. It aimed to determine the feasibility of carrying out a follow-up study of patients suffering from schizophrenia and other functional psychoses in the nine different centers and to examine the course and outcome of patients living in the different cultures.

The second year follow-up of the IPSS had demonstrated that it is feasible to reinterview, assess the mental status of, and collect psychiatric and social history data about a high percentage of patients with functional psychoses 2 years after an initial evaluation in many different cultures, and that there are sharp differences in the course and outcome of schizophrenia in the different centers.[3] At the time of the second-year follow-up, 37 percent (202 out of 543) of schizophrenic patients followed up were psychotic, 31 percent (169 out of 543) were symptomatic but not psychotic, and 32 percent (172 out of 543) were asymptomatic. Ibadan patients clearly had the best course and outcome: 57 percent fell into the best overall outcome group, while only 5 percent fell into the worst overall outcome group. Agra patients had the next best course and outcome for most of the factors considered, including overall outcome.

Aarhus patients had the worst course and outcome: 50 percent were still in the episode of inclusion at the time of the second-year follow-up; 31 percent fell into the worst overall outcome group and only 6 percent into the best group. The other centers varied according to the factor being assessed. In general, Cali and Moscow patients had an intermediate outcome, and Washington, Taipei, and Prague patients a relatively poor outcome.

For all variables considered, the schizophrenic patients in Ibadan, Agra, and Cali (all centers in developing countries) tended to have a better outcome on average than the schizophrenic patients in the other six centers.

Furthermore, it was shown that no single variable, and no combination of a few "key" variables, can explain a large proportion of the variation of any of the course and outcome measures in schizophrenia; in other words, no characteristics of the patient, of the environment, or of the initial manifestations of the disorder considered in isolation would be an effective predictor of the subsequent course and outcome of the illness.

In view of the great potential significance of the IPSS finding, WHO decided to undertake a new study, focused more sharply than the IPSS on the frequency of occurrence, the "natural history" of schizophrenic illnesses, and the factors associated with differences in course and outcome.[4] This study was to be based on more representative patient samples in different cultures. The case-finding strategy designed for the new study consisted in: (i) a prospective surveillance of specified psychiatric, other medical, and social services in a given catchment area in each setting; and (ii) identification of all individuals making a first lifetime contact with such services who exhibited signs and symptoms of a possible schizophrenic illness.*

---

*The alternative design of a cross-sectional community survey, in which a representative *prevalence* sample of cases is identified first and *incidence* is then estimated by attempting to date retrospectively the on-

By extending the case-finding network to include a variety of "helping agencies" in the community (e.g., religious institutions, traditional healers), this strategy was expected to result in a better coverage of the incident cases of the disorder than the first admission method, although patients who never contact *any* agency would still be missed.

Several research techniques that had earlier thrown light on specific facets of the course of schizophrenia were also used. These included the ascertainment of stressful life events prior to the onset of psychotic episodes, the measurement of "expressed emotion" in a key relative, the assessment of the perception of psychotic symptoms by the patient's family, and the evaluation of functional impairments and social disability. It was hoped that the application of these techniques may help to obtain data that could contribute to an explanation of the extraordinary finding of the IPSS that patients in developing countries on the whole have a better outcome than those living in more developed countries.

The total population included in this second major study consisted of 1379 subjects (745 men and 634 women), most of whom were urban residents. With the exception of Ibadan, Cali, and the rural area of Chandigarh, where most patients came from very poor neighborhoods, the socioeconomic status of the patients' neighborhoods and households in the other centers was rated as "average" in comparison with local standards in the majority of cases.

The great majority (86 percent) of the 1218 cases in whom the beginning of the psychotic illness could be dated, had been identified by the case-finding network and assessed within 12 months of the onset of the disorder; in 61 percent this had occurred within 3 months. With regard to the proportion of pa-

---

set of the disorder, was rejected because of (i) low yield of cases per 1000 persons who have to be interviewed; (ii) certainty of missing patients who either died early after the onset of a psychotic illness or migrated out of the area; (iii) exposure of the patients to periods of treatment of varying length and to psychosocial environmental influences that might alter the presenting features of the disorder.

tients with length of previous illness less than 6 months and with 6 months and over, there was no significant difference between the centers in developed and the centers in developing countries.

The study permitted the calculation of incidence of schizophrenia with a "broad" diagnostic definition of the condition (i.e., all included cases except 34 on which insufficient data were available) and with a "restrictive" definition based only on the presence of an initial clinical picture satisfying the criteria for CATEGO class S+.[5] The annual rates were obtained by halving the number of cases identified over 2 years of continuous case-finding and dividing them by the denominator value.

The analysis of incidence was carried out on data from 8 catchment areas in which satisfactory coverage of agencies whom patients might contact was achieved. For the "broad" definition of schizophrenic and related illnesses, the combined rates for males and females varied from 1.5 in Aarhus to 4.2 in observed in Chandigarh (rural area) and amounted to 3.7 and 4.8 per 10,000 respectively. The lowest rates for males (1.8) were found in Aarhus and Honolulu; for females, the lowest rate (1.2) was in Aarhus. The differences across the areas are significant (p 0.001) for males and p 0.0001 for females).

The application of the "restrictive" definition of the CATEGO class S+ resulted in lower combined rates for males and females, ranging from 0.7 in Aarhus to 1.4 in Nottingham. In males, the lowest rate of 0.8 was that in Chandigarh (urban area) and the highest rate of 1.7 was that in Nottingham. In females, the lowest rate (0.5) was found in Aarhus and the highest rate (1.4) in Moscow. The differences in the incidence rates of disorders meeting the CATEGO S+ criteria were not statistically significant in males and only marginally significant (p 0.02) in females. The change in ranges occurring with the application of the "restrictive" definition cannot be explained simply as a loss of the statistical significance of the differences due to a drop in the statistical power to detect such differences in smaller samples: the *actual* values of the incidence rates in the different centers do indeed become more similar to each other. This is contrary to what might be expected to happen as the result of

a mere decrease of individual sample sizes in diagnostically heterogeneous populations and lends support to the notion that the
"central" schizophrenic syndrome may be occurring with approximately equal probability in different populations.

Follow-up examinations of patients, with the full battery of
research instruments (including a follow-up version of the PPHS
and the DAS) were carried out twice, at intervals of 1 year and
2 years following the date of initial screening and inclusion in
the study. In addition to two cross-sections of symptomatology
and one assessment of social disability, the longitudinal, month-
by-month ratings and narrative notes on symptoms and behavior provided the basis for an evaluation of the 2-year (24 +6
months) pattern of course of the disorder. Complete follow-up
data were available on 1,014 (i.e. 74 percent) of the original
1,379 patients. Of those with complete follow-up, 600 subjects
were assessed in centers in developed countries (76 percent of
follow-up coverage) and 414 in centers in developing countries
(71 percent coverage).

A significantly higher percentage (56 percent) of the patients in developing countries exhibited "mild" patterns of
course, compared to the patients in developed countries (39
percent). Also, a significantly higher percentage (40 percent) of
the cases in developed countries had "severe" patterns of course,
compared to the cases in developing countries (24 percent). The
proportions falling into the "intermediate" group were almost
identical in the two settings.

The other studies mentioned above—on the frequency of
life events (Day et al., in press), emotional interaction in families of schizophrenic patients (Leff et al., in press), and the study
of the perception of schizophrenic patients by their families
(Katz et al., in press) have also been successfully completed. Each
of these studies made a methodological contribution and produced new knowledge about schizophrenia. They have involved a large number of investigations and centers in a variety
of countries: the collaboration between these centers established in the course of these studies continued after the studies
were terminated and is undoubtedly a most valuable achieve-
ment of this work.

IMPROVEMENT OF METHODS OF TREATMENT OF SCHIZOPHRENIA

WHO has undertaken considerably less work in this area than in the area of epidemiology. The main reason for this was the profusion of studies on treatment undertaken by researchers all over the world: The likelihood that the addition of WHO's efforts would make a major difference in the increase of knowledge about treatment was slight.

Instead, WHO's emphasis was on linking centers and investigators in different parts of the world, strengthening their position nationally and internationally, and providing stimulation for work on certain priority public health problems. A network of WHO-designated collaborating institutions has thus come into existence: over the years it has grown to become the world's largest network of scientific institutions collaborating in the field of mental health.

On occasion, however, WHO undertook to coordinate research carried out by leading research centers. This usually happened when it was necessary to accumulate data faster or when the design of a study, the attempt to answer a question, required transcultural comparison.

An example of such a study was that on the effects of naloxone on hallucinations in schizophrenia (Pickar et al., 1982).[6] This was a double-blind study of behavioral effects of short-term naloxone hydrochloride administration which was performed in 32 schizophrenic and 26 manic patients in six WHO collaborating centers in the Federal Republic of Germany, India, the Netherlands, Switzerland, the USA, and the USSR. There was a significant naloxone-associated reduction in overall physician-rated symptoms in schizophrenic patients concurrently treated with neuroleptic medication (N = 19) but not in medication-free schizophrenics (N = 13). Physician ratings of auditory hallucinations showed significant naloxone-associated improvement for the total schizophrenic population, while self-ratings of auditory hallucinations showed improvement only in neuroleptic-treated schizophrenics. While further studies are needed to delineate these effects as to clinical significance, they may bear etiological implications for the psychobiology of schizophrenia, including the possibility of synergistic effects of dopamine and endorphin blockage.

Another example, this time of a study undertaken for a different reason, is that of the effects of chlorpromazine on patients suffering from schizophrenia to examine the frequently advanced statement that people in tropical countries can be successfully treated with significantly lower doses of a medicament than people in Europe or other temperate climate countries.

The study could best be undertaken by WHO whose unique position in the field of international health makes it possible to provide coordination and management support to multicentric studies in different countries. The study was a double-blind investigation using a high and low dose of chlorpromazine. It was undertaken in India, Nigeria, Colombia, and Yugoslavia. The results are being analyzed at present. This study is part of a larger effort to produce valid information about the dose-effect relationship prevailing in different parts of the world.[7]

IMPROVEMENT OF KNOWLEDGE ABOUT SCHIZOPHRENIA FACILITATING POLICY FORMULATION AND SERVICE DEVELOPMENT

Two major studies were undertaken by the Organization in this area. The first is a study of disability linked to schizophrenia.

This was undertaken in centers in seven countries. The first phase focused on the development of instruments for the assessment of psychological impairments and specific disabilities in patients suffering from schizophrenic psychoses. These instruments have been applied to assess series of patients and a follow-up study has been undertaken with assessments at 1- and 2-year points after the initial evaluation. It is expected that detailed information will be collected in the course of the study on the nature and extent of impairments and disabilities in the early stages of schizophrenia, and on their prognosis.

The second study was even closer in its focus to primary health care concerns. It began in 1975 as a follow-up to a series of policy decisions concerning the growing commitment to primary health care and the new emphasis and direction in the WHO mental health program, which stresses the public health and social aspects of mental health,[8] and in which the need to develop and evaluate alternative and low-cost methods of mental health care was explicitly recognized.

The technical stimulus for the study came in the form of the specific recommendations of a WHO expert committee that met in 1974 (Technical Report Series on MNH care in developing countries, 1974). The committee, while strongly endorsing the policy of decentralization and integration of services, addressed itself to the "urgent problem . . . of adequate coverage of the population" and advocated the provision of "basic mental health care" by primary health care workers. Since such workers have only limited training and are expected to cope with a number of pressing health problems, the committee stressed the need to limit and define the scope of mental health care provided at this level so that only the fulfillment of "simple and circumscribed tasks" could be expected. Another important recommendation made by the committee was the development of collaboration with nonmedical community agencies, such as teachers, police officers, religious leaders, and local civic associations.

The study took as its starting point the realities of health care provision as it exists in most developing countries and assumed the use of existing health workers, the stimulation of a community response to mental health problems, and a focus on a limited range of priority conditions. It was designed to develop methods required for priority selection, task definition, and training; to determine the feasibility of the committee's recommendations on basic mental health care; and to evaluate the effectiveness of such care.

The organization decided to examine these matters in a collaborative study, since no single developing country would have the resources and expertise to carry out such evaluative research.

Confidence in the possibility of developing well-designed research techniques with crosscultural applicability was provided by the International Pilot Study of Schizophrenia which made significant advances in techniques of translation, reliability testing, rating procedures, and cross-site comparison. That study also demonstrated the feasibility of long-term joint work and fruitful collaboration among research centers in different countries. Some of the methods used in the pilot study and other WHO-coordinated studies were used in this study; two of the centers in the present study participated in the previous efforts.

The collaborative study, especially the practical demonstration that primary health care workers can deliver mental health care to patients suffering from severe mental illness such as schizophrenia at the community level, resulted in a number of effects before the strictly evaluative results became available. The most important effect of this kind was the emergence of a new concept of community psychiatry for developing countries. The fact that primary health care workers are able to carry out mental health actions has served to change attitudes towards disease and health in general as well as towards mental illness; it has served to sensitize workers to important wider psychosocial issues.

An early impact on the attitudes and reactions of administrators and health planners as well as general health care personnel was clearly seen. The initial resistance to dealing with mental health problems that has been observed among general health care personnel soon developed into acceptance. This shift occurred as a result of their participating in and observing the study process rather than because of their objective appraisal of evaluative data. Similar shifts of attitudes occurred among local community leaders, leading to more ready acceptance of mental health care, such as psychiatric clinics and hospitals outside the study areas. Furthermore, neighboring and national health authorities outside the study areas have shown interest in the program.

The study teams have also reported changes in their teaching programs for undergraduate and postgraduate students. Some study team members have already become involved in the planning process at local and national levels in their own countries and have become consultants to other countries. This development has led to the adoption of new approaches to increasing coverage of mental health care through national mental health programs.

CONCLUSION

Schizophrenia is a disease with severe consequences for the individual, his family, community, and country. It presents a number of theoretical and practical questions for which there are no answers. WHO has brought together researchers and institutions from many countries uniting them in an effort to resolve some of the problems posed by schizophrenia. It developed and coordinated a series of investigations, developed methods and mechanisms for international and crosscultural studies, established networks of investigators and institutions collaborating in this area, and produced important contributions to knowledge. The conundrum of schizophrenia is formidable: There is no doubt that the numerous experts and institutions in many lands who have participated in the activities of the WHO mental health program have made an important contribution to its solution.

REFERENCES

1. WHO. Epidemiology of mental disorders. *Technical Report Series*, No. 185, Geneva, 1985.
2. Kramer, M., Sartorius, N., Jablensky, A., & Gulbinat, W. The ICD 9 classification of mental disorders. *Acta Psychiatrica Scandinavica*, 1979, *59*, 241–262.
3. WHO. Schizophrenia: An international follow-up study. New York: Wiley & Sons, 1979.
4. Sartorius, N., Jablensky, A., Korten, A., Ernberg, G., Anker, M., Cooper, J. E., & Day, R. Early manifestations and first contact incidence of schizophrenia in different cultures. *Psychological Medicine*, in press.
5. Wing, J. K., Cooper, J. E., & Sartorius, N. The measurement and classification of psychiatric symptoms. New York: Cambridge University Press, 1974.
6. Pickar, D., et al. Short-term naloxone administration in schizo-

phrenic and manic patients. *Archives of General Psychiatry,* 1982, *39*, 313–319.
7. Sartorius, N. WHO-coordinated studies on the effects of psycho-pharmacological drugs in different populations. In N. Sartrius & H. Helmchen (Eds.) *Multicentric trials.* Basel: Karger, 1981.
8. WHO. Social dimensions of mental health. Geneva, 1981.

Chapter 2

RECENT TRENDS FROM NATURE-NURTURE RESEARCH IN SCHIZOPHRENIA

Fini Schulsinger, M.D.,
Josef Parnas, M.D.,
Hanne Schulsinger, Ph.D.,
Timothy W. Teasdale, Ph.D. &
Sarnoff A. Mednick, M.D., Ph.D.

The purpose of this presentation is to illustrate the justification of studying a possible genetic liability for schizophrenia, and to demonstrate that the effect of possible environmental stressors may vary, depending on genetic liability.

Apart from this, the heuristic value of establishing a genetic liability for schizophrenia is relatively limited. Of course, the very fact that a genetic liability exists justifies research for biological mechanisms being active in the genetic transmission—be they metabolic or neurophysiological.

A better knowledge of the mode of genetic transmission might be very profitable for biological schizophrenia research. The age of onset, the highly varied constellation of symptoms such as autism, cognitive disturbances, paranoid delusions, and hallucinations of various modalities do not speak in favor of a single cause model for schizophrenia. Nor is such a model in accordance with the position of today's psychiatric geneticists who tend to interpret the result of the newer genetic studies of schizophrenia in favor of a polygenetic mode of inheritance.

GENETIC STUDIES

Traditional pedigree studies in schizophrenia have invariably shown that the closer the kinship is between relatives and probands the higher is the risk for schizophrenia in the relatives of the schizophrenic probands. This method has been criticized because a close kinship does not only mean that more genes are in common between the relative and the proband, but also that the resemblance between the environments can be important.

The study of concordance rates for schizophrenia in monozygotic twins, in dizygotic twins, and in ordinary siblings indicate clearly that genetic factors do play a role for schizophrenia.[1]

Also, studies of the prevalence of schizophrenia like disorders in the biological and adoptive relatives of schizophrenic patients who were adopted away to nonbiologically related adoptive families in their early childhood gave definite evidence of the existence of a genetic liability for schizophrenia.[2]

Twin studies, however, have a double function. The fact that concordance for schizophrenia in monozygotic twins very rarely exceeds 50 percent in the major modern twin studies[1] tells us with certainty that genetic factors alone are not responsible for schizophrenia. The studies of monozygotic twins discordant for schizophrenia[3] have indicated a number of individual environmental stressors which—at least in interaction with genetic liability—contribute to the onset of the environmental schizophrenia.

Several environmental researchers have stressed that certain types of rearing and/or certain psychosocial constellations within the family can cause schizophrenia. In some sociological studies correlations between varied disruptive childhood conditions may be correlated to the incidence of schizophrenia. The present author, however, agrees with Gottesman & Shields[4] when they emphasize that though it can not be excluded that certain environmental stressors can produce schizophrenia, such a phenomenon has never been scientifically documented. This is due to the absence of a multidisciplinary approach in many of the most well-known psychosocial schizophrenia studies.[5] These studies do not pay attention to the possibility of interaction between a genetic predisposition towards schizophrenia and the psychosocial stressors.

Such an interaction is not a new invention within the behavioral sciences.

In 1932 the German geneticist Bruno Schulz[6] accounted for the effect of experiential factors on genetic liability for schizophrenia. In a sample of 660 schizophrenic patients he found, among other results, an especially high prevalence of catatonic cases in relation to somatic precipitants.

Manfred Bleuler[7] found in 1941 that a sample of 89 schizophrenic probands who responded favorably to ECT treatment and their relatives who—when compared with relatives of an unselected schizophrenic sample had less conspicuous personalities—were much more seldom schizoid or psychopaths. In cases of schizophrenia these relatives had a much healthier premorbid personality than in the cases of unselected schizophrenics.

Finally, Sigmund Freud[8] in 1937 stated that persons with a strong and healthy "preformed ego" would only develop a neurosis if exposed to very severe traumata, whereas people who had a weak "preformed ego" would develop neurosis if exposed to minimal traumata.

High Risk Studies

A systematic attempt to utilize the way of thinking as demonstrated by the examples from Schulz, Bleuler, and Freud is illustrated by a longitudinal prospective study of children of severely schizophrenic mothers which was initiated in Copenhagen in 1962 by Mednick and Schulsinger.[9] The 207 children

Figure 2-1.   Design of the Project.

High risk children   n = 207
Low risk children   n = 104
±age   15.1 years

1962	♦	1967	♦	1972	♦	1980
INITIAL ASSESSMENT		5-year follow-up		10-year diagnostic follow-up		subsample followup

**Figure 2-1.   Shows the major assessment years in our
study. In addition, we received information
on the subjects from various sources.**

of schizophrenic mothers and their 104 matched low risk controls were between ten and twenty years old, and not yet schizophrenic when the study (continuing in 1986) began. In the
following we shall describe results from four substudies on the
same sample:

1)   An analysis of pregnancy and birth complications dis-
     tributed over diagnostic outcome in 1972–1974.

2)   An analysis of institutional care during the first 5 years
     of life, and the diagnostic outcome in 1972–1974.

3)   An analysis of premorbid behavior until the 1962 as-
     sessment, and diagnostic outcome in 1972–1974.

4)   Data from a study carried out 1979–1980 in order to
     test a hypothesis on the nature of what is genetically
     transmitted, and what is not.

OBSTETRICAL DATA

Detailed midwife reports were rated on a 0–4 weighted rating scale for specific complications. This scale was developed
with the assistance of professor Frits Fuchs of the Department

of Gynecological Obstetrics at Cornell University Medical School. The individual scores could be utilized to create three different global scores of pregnancy and birth complications.

1) Frequency score
2) Severity score
3) Total score

The total score was derived by adding all the individual weighted scores, and the total score correlated highly with the other scores. Figure 2-2 shows the total scale scores for the four

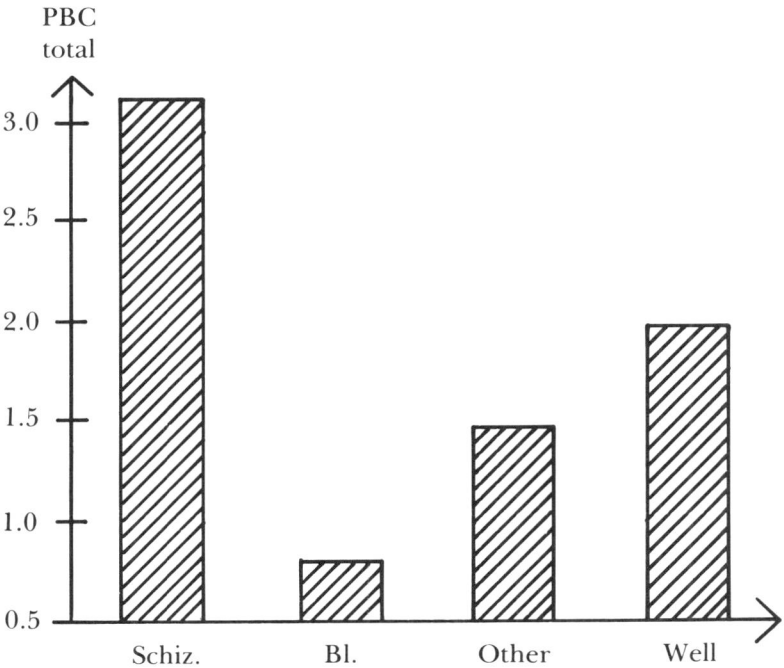

Figure 2-2. Pregnancy and birth complications in high-risk group.

diagnostic groups: schizophrenia, borderline schizophrenia, other diagnoses, or well. The schizophrenic group had significantly higher complication scores than the borderline group. The mean values for the well group do not differ significantly from either those of the schizophrenics or those of the borderlines. In fact the mean values for the well group lie close to the midpoint between these two pathological groups. The majority of the schizophrenics (67 percent) experienced some form or other of complication, which means that our results do not come from very few schizophrenics suffering a tremendous amount of severe complications. These results which are reported[10] will be discussed eventually.

BEHAVORIAL PRECURSORS OF SCHIZOPHRENIA SPECTRUM

During the first assessment of our subjects from 1962–1964 we collected information on the subjects' behavior from infancy up to the time of assessment. We interviewed their rearing parents or rearing agencies. All the subjects were interviewed during the assessment, and all the investigators involved completed an adjective checklist on the subjects. Finally we got very detailed information from the classmasters about the subjects' achievements and behavior in school.

Figure 2-3 demonstrates the overall results from the study of premorbid behavioral characteristics within the schizophrenia spectrum. Part of the information is retrospective, as for example the early childhood factors where we find that schizophrenia spectrum, i.e. schizophrenia and borderline schizophrenia, exhibited passivity and poor attention according to the parental descriptions. School behavior was retrospective to some extent, but for the majority of the subjects the information was actually present. We found that schizophrenia spectrum subjects in school were more isolated and rejected by others, and they were more sensitive. In addition they were characterized by poor affect control, they were more easily upset, and more liable to contain their distress for a longer time than the com-

Figure 2-3. Behavioral Precursors of Schizophrenia Spectrum.

Early childhood	passivity
	poor concentration
School behavior	rejected by others
	poor affect control*
Clinical assessment	(15 years of age)
	formal thought disorder
	defective emotional rapport

*This item discriminated schizophrenics from borderline schizophrenics.

parison groups. With regard to this item, the schizophrenics were significantly worse than the borderlines which was the only significant difference between these two parts of the schizophrenia spectrum. The clinical assessment items were nonretrospective and they comprised cognitive as well as emotional items as premorbid discriminators.

As a preliminary conclusion of the behavioral precursor study, which is described in detail,[11] we can state that our results seem to point toward a basic behavioral relationship between schizophrenia and borderline schizophrenia. Both disorders were characterized by premorbidly defective emotional rapport and formally disturbed cognition. Preschizophrenics, however, tended to display more attention deficit and exhibited poor affective control. In their psychopathological picture both disorders exhibit fundamental schizophrenic symptoms but of course to a different degree. The distinction between them, however, relies mainly on the intensity of accessory psychotic symptoms such as hallucinations and delusions. This study of behavioral precursors substantiate Eugen Bleuler's concept of schizophrenia as a disorder essentially characterized by formally disturbed cognition and defective emotional rapport: The disease is characterized by a specific type of alteration of thinking, feeling, and relation to the external world that appears nowhere else in this particular fashion. Hallucinations and delusions are partial phenomena of the most varied diseases. Their presence is often helpful in making the diagnosis of a psychosis, but not in diagnosing the presence of schizophrenia.

As the fundamental symptoms can be traced premorbidly, we find Bleuler's concept of schizophrenia as a development, rather than as a disease process striking a healthy person, is substantiated by our results.

INSTITUTIONALIZATION

The basic advantage of the prospective, high risk design is that it makes it possible to find out which environmental factors might be correlated to the differences in clinical outcome. Michael Rutter[12] concluded his review of the consequences of deprivation in childhood by endorsing Caldwell's recommendation that the future should fulfill three criteria, namely: 1) taking genetic factors into account, 2) employing stringently defined measures of stress, and 3) focusing upon specific psychopathological outcome variables. We have tried to analyze the history of institutionalization in relation to the clinical outcome within and outside the schizophrenia spectrum in our sample of children of severely schizophrenic mothers. We proposed, with respect to genetic loading, that schizophrenics and borderline schizophrenics share a similar genetic predisposition that is more severe than that of those high risk individuals who remain mentally healthy. Operationally, this means that we hypothesize that the age of onset of maternal schizophrenia should be lower among schizophrenics and borderline schizophrenics than among high risk individuals who remain healthy. With respect to the environmental factors we have suggested that it is in particular the schizophrenics themselves rather than borderlines who have premorbidly experienced the most stressful conditions. Operationally this means that schizophrenics should have spent more time in institutions during the first 5 years of life than did other diagnostic outcome groups.

Table 2-1 presents means and standard deviations for each of the three independent variables as a function of diagnoses in the high risk group. In this study we have also included a group of all the other diagnoses apart from schizophrenia, borderline schizophrenia, and no mental illness. The three variables are: Mother's age at first hospitalization (MAH), the number of months spent in institution during the first 5 years of life (INS), and finally the number of months spent with the schizophrenic mother during the first 5 years of life (CM). Both the schizophrenics and borderlines have mothers whose age at first hospitalization was significantly younger than those of the no mental illness group. The "other diagnoses" group occupied a middle position.

With respect to institutionalization (INS) the schizophrenics have experienced significantly more through the first 5 years of life than have the borderlines, who in turn fall significantly above the "other diagnoses" as well as the "no mental illness" group on this variable. In the case of contact with the mother (CM) the schizophrenics had significantly less contact with the mothers during the first 5 years of life than had both the other diagnoses and no mental illness groups which do not differ significantly from each other. These three variables can be expected to be heavily intercorrelated, as was found.

An analysis of covariance of institutionalization corrected for mother's age at first hospitalization and for contact with the mother showed that institutionalization significantly keeps its effect. If we entered mother's age at hospitalization and institutionalization as covariates for contact with the mother, the four diagnostic groups did not differ significantly. Thus, contact with the mother may only have significance for later psychopathology in the child to the extent it indirectly reflects the degree of genetic loading the child has inherited and/or the amount of time spent in institutions. A detailed report on institutionalization has been published.[13]

CEREBRAL VENTRICULAR SIZE WITHIN THE SCHIZOPHRENIA SPECTRUM

A number of studies over the last 3 decades indicate that chronic schizophrenia is associated with cerebral ventricular en-

Table 2-1. Predictor Variables as a Function of Diagnosis (High Risk Group only)

	Schizophrenics N = 13		Borderline Schizophrenics N = 29		Other Diagnoses N = 76		No Mental Illness N = 55		ANOVA	P
	mean	s.d.	mean	s.d.	mean	s.d.	mean	s.d.	F	
MAH (age)	27.7	5.4	29.5	8.3	32.1	8.2	34.5	8.3	3.86	.011
INS (months)	22.2	22.8	10.8	16.0	4.1	10.6	2.4	7.6	11.33	<.001*
CM (months)	32.5	23.5	41.6	21.0	50.1	17.2	50.3	18.1	4.66	.004*

*In view of the skew of these two variables we have repeated the analyses using a non parametric test (Kruskal-Wallis).

For INS the corresponding probability is <.001 and for CM .003.

largement. The NIHM studies of twins discordant for schizophrenia showed that the schizophrenic twins had more soft
neurological signs than had the healthy co-twins. Other studies,
for example by Max Pollock and coworkers, have shown that
siblings of schizophrenics have less neurological deficit than had
the schizophrenics themselves. As described above, we, and
many others, have shown that schizophrenics have suffered
more pregnancy and birth complications than the other high
risk children. Taking into consideration also that the Ameri-
can-Danish adoption studies[2] have demonstrated that schizophrenia and borderline schizophrenia appears among the
biological relatives of the same schizophrenic index probands,
we forwarded the hypothesis that the genetically transmitted
condition is not schizophrenia itself but borderline schizophrenia. Real schizophrenia then is a complicated (frequently neu-
rologically complicated) form of borderline schizophrenia. Our
concept of borderline schizophrenia corresponds with the DSM-
111 schizotypal personality disorder.

In order to test this bold hypothesis we studied from
1979–1980 a subgroup of the total high risk sample consisting
of 10 schizophrenics, 10 borderlines, and 16 no mental illness
cases, as diagnosed in our 1972-assessment during which diagnoses were made as a consensus between two of three diagnostic instruments: a clinical diagnosis, the Current And Past
Psychopathology Scale (CAPPS), or the Present State Examination (PSE) 9th edition. In 1979–1980 these 36 subjects were
clinically reassessed by the same clinical interviewer, and the
subjects were also examined with a 1010 EMI-scanner. We used
the same method of measurement as reported by Weinberger
and his colleagues from the United States.

There were no significant differences in the third ventricle
width or the ventricle-brain-ratio (VBR) as a function of the
1972 consensus or even the 1972 clinical diagnoses. However,
the clinical diagnoses made in 1980 had changed to some extent from the clinical diagnoses in 1972. Two of the schizophrenias had turned into borderlines, one of the borderlines
had turned into schizophrenia, one into no mental illness, and
one into other psychiatric disorders. Comparisons based on the
1980 diagnoses showed that schizophrenics had the largest third

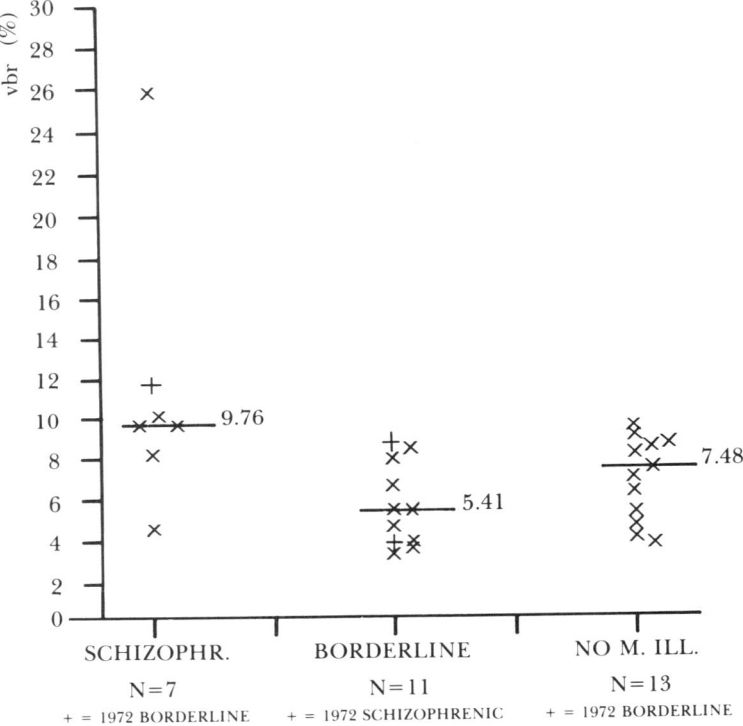

Figure 2-4.   VBR by 1980 diagnosis.

ventricles. Figure 4 showed that ventricular size as measured by the VBR was the largest for the schizophrenics and the smallest for the borderlines, with the no mental illness group in between. No relationship was found between ventricular size and the age of the subject, length of psychiatric hospitalization, drug treatment, or electroconvulsive treatment.

We examined the relationship between ventricular size in 1980 and the pregnancy-birth complication data obtained as part of the initial 1962-assessment. We found significant associations between enlarged ventricles in adulthood and signs of pregnancy at birth. There was also a modest correlation between maturity the width of third ventricle and a global rating of perinatal complications. For further information see.[14]

CONCLUSION

It is an almost insuperable task to report results from more than 20 year prospective work with this group of children of schizophrenic mothers and their controls. In the references[10, 11, 13, 14, 15, 16] detailed descriptions and discussions about methodology and about the concepts of the various parts of the schizophrenia spectrum may be found. What we have tried to show is *one* development within the genetics of schizophrenia: The utilization of genetic knowledge to facilitate the study of possible environmental effects. We have seen that the clinical outcome of the children of severely schizophrenic mothers to some extent may depend on obstetrical complications, and on institutional care. We have seen that premorbidly there is a great overlap between the components of the schizophrenia spectrum. We have also seen that differences in ventricular size to some extent might be a reflection of differences in environment. We believe that prospective studies of populations at a high risk for schizophrenia are the most powerful way of studying the interactions between heredity and environment. First, it is not too burdened by the doubtful reliability of retrospective information. Second, the value of following the same specific individuals over time is a strong advantage as demonstrated with the diagnostic changes over time in the cerebral ventricle study. Third, the high risk design not only permits us to study the effect of a defined stressor upon various levels of genetic risk, but also the effects of various degrees of the same stressor upon one defined genetic risk level. Finally, the high risk design provides us with the best possible controls: those high risk subjects who do not become schizophrenics in spite of the genetic risk.

This approach in nature-nurture research, which for generations has been a matter of course within botanical, agricultural, and zoological research, also seems to have potentials within the human behavioral sciences.

REFERENCES

1. Gottesman I. I., & Shields, J. Schizophrenia and genetics: A twin study vantage point. New York: Academic Press, 1972.

2. Kety, S. S., Rosenthal, D., Wender, P.H., et al. Mental illness in the biological and adoptive relatives of adopted individuals who became schizophrenic. In *Genetic Research in Psychiatry* R. Fieve, D. Rosenthal, & Brill H. (Eds). Baltimore, MD: Johns Hopkins University Press, 1975.

3. Pollin, W., & Stabenau, J. R., Biological, psychological, and historical differences in a series of monozygotic twins discordant for schizophrenia. *Journal Psychiatric Research*, 1968, *6*, Suppl 1:317–332.

4. Gottesman, I. I., & Shields, J Rejoinder: Toward optimal arousal and away from original din. *Schizophrenia Bulletin*, 1976, 2:447–453.

5. Lidz, T., Fleck, S., Cornelison, A. Schizophrenia and the family. New York: International University Press, 1965.

6. Schulz, B. Zur Erbpathologie der Schizophrenen. *Zeitschrift gesellschaft für Neurologie und Psychiatrie*, 1932, *143*:175–293.

7. Bleuler M: Das Wesen der Schizophrenie nach schockbehandlung. *Zeitschr ges Neurol und Psychiatr*, 1941, *173*:553–597.

8. Freud S: Die endliche und die unendliche Analysen. In Ges Werke, London: Imago Publishing Co., Ltd, Vol. 16:64, 1937.

9. Mednick, S. A., & Schulsinger, F. A longitudinal study of children with a high risk for schizophrenia: A preliminary report. In *Methods and Goals in Human Behavior Genetics*. S. Vanderberg, (Ed.) New York: Academic Press, 1965.

10. Parnas, J., Schulsinger, F., Teasdale, T. W., et al. Perinatal complications and clinical outcome within the schizophrenia spectrum. *British Journal of Psychiatry*, 140:416–420, 1982.

11. Parnas, J., Schulsinger, F., Schulsinger, H., et al. Behavioral precursors of schizophrenia spectrum. *Archives of General Psychiatry*, 1982, *39*:658–664.

12. Rutter, M. Maternal deprivation reassessed. Hammondworths. Penguin Books Ltd., 1981.

13. Parnas, J., Teasdale, T. W., & Schulsinger, H. Institutional rearing and diagnostic outcome in children of schizophrenic mothers. *Archives of General Psychiatry*, 1985, *42*:762–769.

14. Schulsinger, F., Parnas, J., Petersen, E.T., et al. Cerebral ventricular size in the offspring of schizophrenic mothers: A preliminary study. *Archives of General Psychiatry*, 1984, *41*:602–606.

15. Mednick, S. A., & Schulsinger, F. Studies of children at high risk for schizophrenia. In *Schizophrenia: The first ten Dean Award Lectures.* Edited by MSS Information Service, New York: 245–293, 1973.

16. Schulsinger, H. A ten-year follow-up of children of schizophrenic mothers: Clinical assessment. *Acta Psychiatrica Scandinavica,* 1976, *53*:371.

Chapter 3

GENES AND VIRUSES IN SCHIZOPHRENIA

The Retrovirus/Transposon Hypothesis

Timothy J. Crow

Discussions of the etiology of schizophrenia cannot avoid the question of a genetic contribution. Such a component is suggested by twin[1] and adoption[2-4] study evidence. Although there are still some dissenters,[5-8] the adoption studies establish at least that there is a genetic influence. However, the nature of this component remains obscure. Problems for a "pure" genetic hypothesis are the extent of discordance in monozygotic twins (the highest figure reported in the recent studies reviewed by Gottesman is 58 percent), the fact that the onset often occurs after some years of normal function, and that the disease is associated with a fertility disadvantage but retains a high prevalence. These considerations encourage the search for environmental as well as genetic contributions of etiology.

BACKGROUND AND THE CONTAGION HYPOTHESIS

A viral hypothesis of schizophrenia was first clearly enunciated by Menninger[9] and Goodall[10] following the influenza pandemic of 1918 and the encephalitis lethargica epidemic which occurred not long afterwards (and may possibly have been related).[11] Schizophrenialike psychoses were seen in association with both these diseases and have since been reported as occasional concomitants of viral illness and encephalitis of presumed viral etiology.[12, 13] Thus it might be suggested that schizophrenia is either an unusual reaction to a known virus (as may have been observed in the 1918 influenza epidemic) or is caused by a neurotropic virus which has yet to be identified. The role of genes in etiology could be accounted for on the basis of a gene-infectious agent interaction for which there is evidence in the case of poliomyelitis and tuberculosis.

Although it is widely believed that the prevalence of schizophrenia is constant with respect to time and place, this view has recently been contested. Thus Torrey[14] assessed the evidence for significant geographical variations and Hare[15] reviewed records that suggest an increase in incidence in the course of the nineteenth century. Such findings are compatible with a viral hypothesis. Findings and hypothesis together generate the prediction that transmission is sometimes horizontal.

The concept of psychosis as a contagious disease was first considered in reports of cases of folie a deux.[16-18] That horizontal transmission is of more general, perhaps virological, significance was mooted[19] following examination of some anomalies, from a genetic viewpoint, in the data from family studies of schizophrenia. Thus concordance rates have generally been reported as higher in dyzygotic twin pairs than in siblings, and higher in the same sex that in opposite sex pairs of relatives. These findings are consistent with the view that proximity to an affected individual, in addition to genetic predisposition, is relevant to disease onset, as also are the findings of an analysis of time of onset of illness in monozygotic twin pairs.[20] Further grist to the mill of the contagion theory is a brief report from Moscow[21] that first episodes of illness are more likely to occur in individuals who are living in proximity to (unrelated) patients with the disease.

AGE OF ONSET IN SIBLING PAIRS

Thus that schizophrenia is a disease which is horizontally transmitted between individuals with a genetic predisposition

could not be ruled out.[19] However, the theory can be more in-
cisively examined in pairs of siblings with the disease. If one
member of a sibship already has the disease, some of his siblings are likely to have the genetic disposition and they will also
be exposed to someone with the disease. Thus age of onset of
illness in pairs of siblings may illuminate the contagious issue.

In an analysis of five sets of data[22] it was found that age of
onset is highly correlated (r = 0.59 to 0.86) between siblings.
Moreover, there is a consistent tendency (p 0.0005 for the five
studies taken together) for age of onset to be younger in the
younger sibling (Figure 3-1). This could be because (i) the illness is diagnosed earlier when it is already known to be present
in the family (the "early detection" hypothesis), (ii) the disease
is horizontally transmitted (the "contagion" hypothesis), or (iii)
an excess of early onsets in younger siblings is included when
the data are collected at the time of onset of illness in one sibling rather than at the end of the lifetime risk period (the "ascertainment bias" hypothesis).

The first two hypotheses can be distinguished from the
third by analyzing the time (i.e., the order) of onset of illness.

These hypotheses predict that the age shift (to younger age
in younger sibling) will be seen in pairs in which the elder sibling is ill first—this is the essence of the early detection explanation, and the contagion hypothesis predicts that the age shift
will be seen, whichever twin is ill first (unless a long latent period is present). The "ascertainment bias" (the third) hypothesis
predicts, on the contrary, that the age shift will be seen only in
those pairs in which the younger sibling is ill first because the
bias postulated is that an excess of early and first onsets and a
deficit of late onsets in younger siblings will be included. This is
what is observed (Figure 3-2).

The finding suggests rather strongly that ascertainment
bias is present and that when this is removed, by excluding
first onsets in younger siblings, no age shift is present, although
the correlation between ages of onset remains (r = 0.73). While
the findings are not perhaps a decisive rejection of the contagion theory (for example, it could be suggested that if a latent
period is present which is of similar magnitude to the difference in dates of birth in siblings, the age shift expected on the

contagion hypothesis would not be seen in the elder sibling-ill first pairs) they provide little support for it. Ascertainment bias rather than contagion appears to be the likely explanation of the age shift in the total sample. In general, the data lead one to believe that "environmental factors" which are shared by the siblings are not relevant to age of onset. If such factors (e.g., childhood viral infections, loss of a parent, even the psychological impact of onset of illness in a sibling) were significant a shift toward younger age of onset in younger sibling would be seen in the elder sibling-ill first pairs. Age of onset thus is determined by genetic (or at least prenatal) rather than environmental factors. Some other explanation than horizontal transmission is required for the correlation between ages of onset in siblings. If the data can be relied upon, it appears that whatever it is that leads to schizophrenia is present like a clock, from before birth, ticking away to wreak its pathological effects at a predestined time in the life of the affected individual.

RETROVIRUSES/TRANSPOSONS AND SEASON OF BIRTH

That the data do not exclude a prenatal influence draws attention to the well established season of birth effect—the tendency for individuals who later become schizophrenic to have been born in the winter months.[23-26] The observations suggest that in some patients a critical event occurs at an early stage of development. One possibility is that a virus with a very long latency becomes established before birth; such latency might depend upon the genes of the host. An alternative, and perhaps simpler, hypothesis to account for the postulated role of both gene and virus is that the pathogen is either a virus that becomes integrated in the human genome or an element that can transpose to a site within the genome at which it exerts its pathogenic effects. Such an agent would exist as a "provirus" within the genome and could be passed from one generation to the next. According to this view, the disease occurs either as a result of inheritance from an affected or predisposed parent or as a result of an integration or transposition event occurring early in ontogeny. The season of birth effect would be relevant

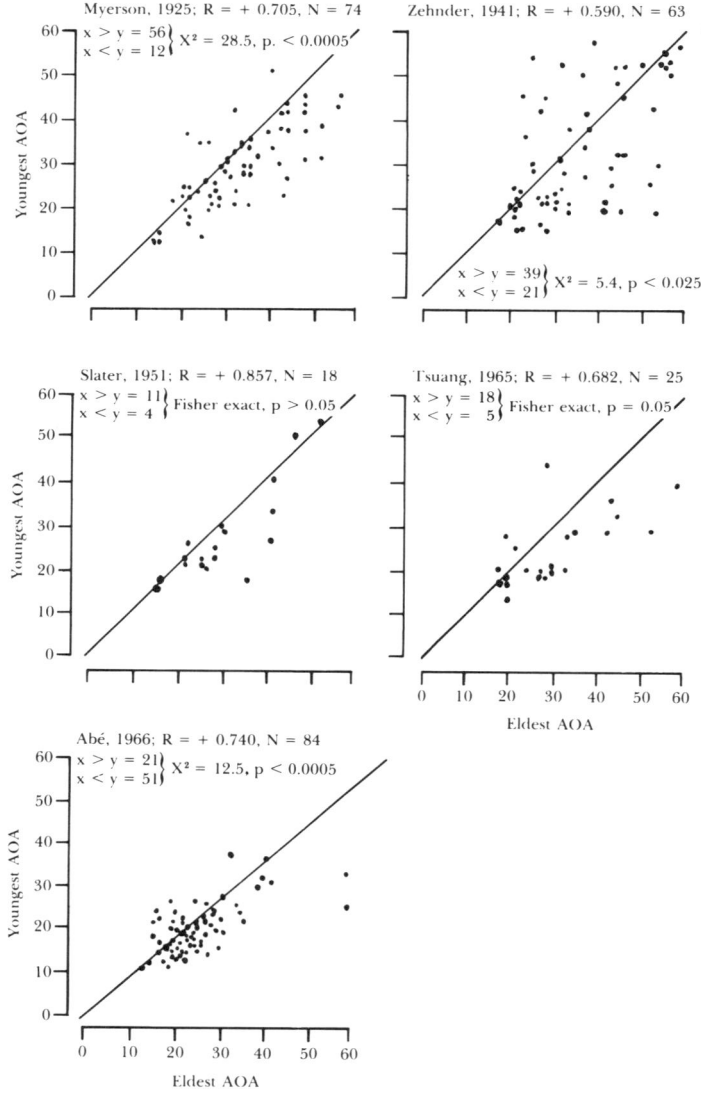

Figure 3-1.   Age on first admission (AOA) to psychiatric hospital in pairs of siblings with schizophrenia (Crow & Done, submitted).

The data are taken from 5 studies:
Myerson, A. Inheritance of Mental
Disorders. Williams & Wilkins,
Baltimore, 1928; Zehnder, von M.
Monat.f.Psychiat.u.Neurol. (Berlin), *103*
231, 1941; Slater, E. Psychotic and Neurotic
illness in twins.
MRC Special Report series No.278. HMSO,
London, 1953; Tsuang, M.T. Ph.D. thesis,
University of London, 1965; Abe, K.
Psychiat. Neurol. (Basel) 151, 276 (1966).
Correlation coefficients (r values) are given
in each case and a p-value calculated
against the null hypothesis that age of onset
will be the same in elder and younger
siblings.

to the latter but not the former. It is of particular interest that in the Danish adoption sample Kinney and Jacobsen[27] observed, the excess of winter births was present particularly in those who lacked a family history of the disease.

The hypothesis that the disease is due to a pathogen integrated in "proviral" form in the human genome (the retrovirus/transposon hypothesis) encounters two difficulties:

(i)   that the site of integration must be constant (and perhaps expressed in brain) for the disease to be consistent in its manifestations, and

(ii)   the low rate of concordance in monozygotic twins.

CEREBRAL DOMINANCE AND PROTO-ONCOGENES

A solution to these difficulties may be found in the role of cerebral dominance. Flor-Henry[28] reported that the schizophreniform psychoses of temporal lobe epilepsy were almost always associated with a focus in the left hemisphere. He and others have suggested that schizophrenia itself is in some sense

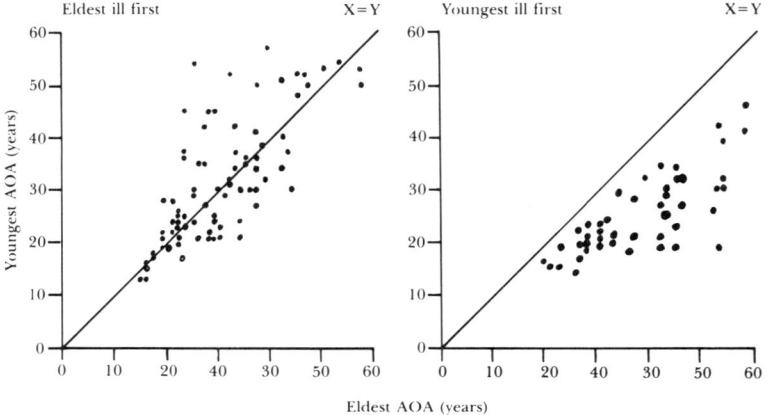

**Figure 3-2. Age of onset in pairs of siblings divided
according to whether the elder or younger
sibling is ill first. The sample (n = 170) is
taken from data in the 5 studies included
in Figure 1, from pairs where order of
onset could be determined; pairs are
excluded when the illness occurred in both
siblings in the same year (from Crow &
Done, submitted).**

a disease of the dominant hemisphere and two recent postmor-
tem brain studies[29, 30] give support to this concept. For the viral
hypothesis this notion provokes the awkward question of how a
virus could be confined to one hemisphere, and also raises the
issue of the cerebral basis of dominance and its genetic determination.

That these issues indeed are relevant to schizophrenia is
rather strongly suggested by Boklage[31] reanalysis of the twin
series of Slater and Gottesman, and Shields, by the handedness
of the individual members of each monozygotic pair. Boklage
found that 92 percent of MZ pairs were concordant for schizophrenia when both twins were right-handed (the 2-RH pairs)
but only 25 percent of pairs were concordant when one or more
member was not right-handed (1-2 NRH pairs). An explana-

tion of these findings requires an account of the genetics of dominance including why monozygotic twins are not always concordant for handedness. Perhaps the simplest account is that of Annett[32] who suggests that handedness is determined by a right-shift factor, dominantly inherited. When this factor is present the individual is left-hemisphere dominant and right-handed; when it is absent which hemisphere shall be dominant is determined by a random process. On this, and probably most other theories, Boklage's findings suggest that the genetics of cerebal dominance and schizophrenia are interrelated. Further, the findings provide one possible explanation for discordance for schizophrenia in twins—when the dominance factor is absent, the substrate on which genetic transmission depends is lost, and handedness is randomly determined.

The presence or absence of the right-shift factor (or dominance gene) has morphological effects in the brain. Geschwind and colleagues[33] have described how the left planum temporale in the human brain is generally more prominent than the right, the asymmetry being more frequent in right-handed individuals. Presumably such asymmetry is due to differential growth and could result from the presence of a growth factor which in right-handed subjects is activated preferentially in the left hemisphere.

Such a concept is relevant to the integrated virus/transposon hypothesis. The retroviruses, for example, have an affinity for growth factors or "proto-oncogenes." If, therefore, we assume that cerebral dominance is determined by the presence of a gene (the dominance gene) it might be further suggested that the retrovirus or transposon postulated as the cause of psychosis has an affinity for this growth factor or proto-oncogene. Retrovirus/transposon integration at the site of the dominance gene could explain the apparent selectivity of the disease for the left hemisphere.[34]

The simplest version of this hypothesis predicts that schizophrenia will be a disease confined to right-handed people. This is not the case. Surveys of populations of psychiatric patients do not show striking deviations from the normal population is handedness patterns,[35] although there is evidence[36] that left-handers who develop schizophrenia have a milder form of the disease. Nor is discordance for schizophrenia in monozygotic twins always associated with discordance for handedness. Thus Luchins et al.[37] examined handedness in 10 pairs of monozygotic twins selected for discordance for schizophrenia, and found that 7 of these pairs were both right-handed. A possible explanation is that in these cases the disease is acquired (perhaps at an early stage of development) rather than inherited from an affected or predisposed parent. Some support for this is the observation that in each of these 7 twin pairs the individual who later became schizophrenic weighed less at birth.

The association between the dominant hemisphere and psychosis in the absence of a clear relationship between handedness and schizophrenia suggests the possibility that handedness is a quantitative rather than qualitative trait and that perhaps the factor that causes increased growth in the (L) hemisphere in right-handed individuals is not absent in ambidextrous or left-handed individuals but merely more symmetrically localized. This would explain a general tendency for the disease to be in the left hemisphere (since most people are right-handed) without a deficit of cases in left-handers. The diminished severity of the illness in left-handers could be due to a greater degree of flexibility of cerebral organization in these individuals.

MECHANISMS OF TRANSMISSION OF PSYCHOSES

That there is a relationship between major affective disorder (manic-depressive illness) and schizophrenia is hinted by the observation that intermediate states (e.g., schizo-affective psychoses) are commonly observed and no satisfactory dividing line can be drawn between the two major psychoses.[38] Furthermore, season of birth effects closely similar to those in schizophrenia are seen in groups of individuals with manic-depressive psychoses,[24] and there is some evidence[34] that there is an excess of schizophrenia among the children of patients with affective illness. Such family findings are in conflict with the conventional view that the two psychoses are genetically independent and raise the possibility that genetic changes take place between one generation and the next. Changes in this type are easier to understand if in the psychoses we are dealing with a proto-oncogene or growth factor that can be modified by a retrovirus or other type of mobile genetic element. Some findings in family studies imply that anomalies of cerebral dominance have an influence on the incidence of psychosis. Thus there may be a deficit of left handers amongst the parents of schizophrenics[39] and an excess amongst the relatives of patients with manic-depressive illness.[40] Perhaps a balanced polymorphism with respect to handedness is maintained by evolutionary advantages against which are offset the disadvantages associated with psychoses. Maybe the advantage of a polymorphism with respect to cerebral dominance is related in some way to the peculiarly human capacity for speech, and the persistence of the psychosis gene is due to its ability to confer flexibility on the determinants of dominance. Such a view is compatible with the concept that psychosis itself is related to genes associated with particular advantages,[41-43] although it remains to be shown that they have survival value. If the psychosis genes are associated with compensatory biological advantages this could explain why it persists in spite of the decreased fertility that results from psychosis itself.

If no such advantage exists, then some form of horizontal transmission must be postulated to explain the persistence of the psychoses. Analysis of age of onset of siblings[22] does not exclude prenatal horizontal transmission. Retroviral infection in utero is one possibility but another is transposition of a mobile genetic element. Such transpositions have been found to be temperature dependent;[44] this could be relevant to the season of birth effect. Of perhaps even greater interest is the possibility that transposable elements can spread more rapidly than conventional genes in a sexually reproducing population and that they may do so in spite of deleterious effects on the host organism.[45] There is evidence[46] that the I and P transposable elements have spread recently within drosophila populations. The possibility that a similar spread of a mobile genetic element in the human population occurs as a result of transposition events related to sexual reproduction deserves consideration. This could account for temporal variations in the incidence of psychosis.[15]

We may conclude the following:

1. Although a genetic contribution to psychosis is strongly suggested by twin and adoption studies, a simple genetic theory of schizophrenia encounters the problems that (i) concordance in MZ twins falls short of 100 percent, (ii) age of onset is often well into adult life, (iii) the mode of inheritance is obscure, and (iv) the disease persists even though it confers a fertility disadvantage.

2. The hypothesis that schizophrenia is a virus disease to which a genetically predisposed subgroup of the population is susceptible generates the prediction that horizontal transmission occurs. An analysis of age of onset in pairs of siblings with the disease indicates that horizontal transmission probably does not occur at the time of onset of illness or at any time in postnatal life.

3. The alternative hypothesis is proposed that schizophrenia is due to a retrovirus or transposon which becomes integrated in the human genome. According to this concept, the "psychosis gene" is acquired either from an affected or predisposed parent or by an integration/transposition event occuring early in ontogeny. If such integration/transposition events are temperature dependent this provides an explanation for the season of birth effect, and the observation that seasonality of birth occurs particularly in those without a family history. If the retrovirus/transposon integrates at a site close to the gene which determines cerebral dominance this could explain the apparent affinity of the disease for the left cerebral hemisphere.

4. The occurrence of season of birth effects in both manic-depressive psychosis and schizophrenia, a tendency for the former to be succeeded in later generations by the latter, and the existence of intermediate states, suggest that the etiologies of these illnesses are more closely related than is often supposed.

5. The persistence of psychotic illness at a high prevalence in spite of its deleterious effects on fertility indicates either that the psychosis gene is associated with biological advantages (per-

haps related to the evolution of cerebral dominance and creativity) or that horizontal transmission occurs at a point before birth, for example by spread of a transposable element in the course of sexual reproduction (e.g., at meiosis).

REFERENCES

1. Gottesman, I.I. Schizophrenia and genetics: Where are we? Are you sure? In L.C. Wynne, R.L. Cromwell, & S. Matthysse (Eds.), *The nature of schizophrenia*. New York: Wiley, 1978.
2. Heston, L.L. Psychiatric disorders in foster home reared children of schizophrenic mothers. *British Journal of Psychiatry*, 1966, *112*, 819–825.
3. Karlsson, J.L. The rate of schizophrenia in foster-reared close relatives of schizophrenic index cases. *Biological Psychiatry*, 1970, *2*, 285–290.
4. Kety, S.S., Rosenthal, D., Wender, P.H., Schulsinger, F., & Jacobsen, B. The biologic and adoptive families of individuals who became schizophrenic: Prevalence of mental illness and other characteristics. In L.C. Wynne, R.L. Cromwell, & S. Matthysse (Eds.), *The nature of schizophrenia*. New York: Wiley, 1978.
5. Lidz, T., Blatt S. & Cook, B. Critique of the Danish-American studies of the of the adopted away offspring of schizophrenic parents. *American Journal of Psychiatry*, 1981, *138*, 1063–1068.
6. Lidz, T., Blatt, S. Critique of the Danish-American studies of the biological and adoptive relatives of adoptees who became schizophrenic. *American Journal of Psychiatry*, 1983 *140*, 426–434.
7. Pope, H.G., Jonas, J.M., Cohen, B.M., & Lipinski, J.F. Failure to find evidence of schizophrenia in first-degree relatives of schizophrenic probands. *American Journal of Psychiatry*, 1982, *139*, 826–828.
8. Abrams, R., & Taylor, M.A. The genetics of schizophrenia: A reassessment using modern criteria. *American Journal of Psychiatry*, 1983, *140*, 171–175.
9. Menninger, K.A. The schizophrenia syndrome as a product of acute infectious disease. *Archives of Neurological Psychiatry*, 1928, *20*, 464–481.

10. Goodall, E. The exciting cause of certain states, at present classified under "schizophrenia" by psychiatrists, may be infection. *Journal of Mental Science*, 1932, *78*, 746–755.
11. Ravenholt, R.T., & Foege, W.H. 1918 Influenza, encephalitis lethargica, Parkinsonism, *Lancet*, 1982, *ii*, 860–864.
12. Torrey, E.F., & Petersen, M.R. The viral hypothesis of schizophrenia. *Schizophrenia Bulletin*, 1976, *2*, 136–146.
13. Crow, T.J. Viral causes of psychiatric disease. *Postgraduate Medical Journal*, 1978, *54*, 763–767.
14. Torrey, E.F. Schizophrenia and civilization. New York: Jason Aronson, 1980.
15. Hare, E.H. Was insanity on the increase? *British Journal of Psychiatry*, 1983, *142*, 439–455.
16. Hofbauer, B. Infectio Psychica. *Osterreichische Medicinische Wochenschrift*, 1846, *39*, 1184–1188.
17. Beillarger, L. Example de contagion d'un delire monomanique. *La Moniteur des Hospitaux*, 1857, *45*, 353–354.
18. Wollenberg, R. Ueber psychische infection. *Archiv. für Psychiatrie*, 1889, *20*, 62–88.
19. Crow, T.J. Is schizophrenia an infectious disease? *Lancet*, 1983, *i*, 173–175.
20. Abe, K. The morbidity rate and environmental influence in monozygotic co-twins of schizophrenics, *British Journal of Psychiatry*, 1969 *115*, 519–531.
21. Kasanetz, E.F. Tecnica per investigare il ruolo di fattori ambientale sulla genesi della schizofrenia. *Rivista di Psicologie Analitica*, 1979, *10*, 193–202.
22. Crow, T.J., & Done, D.J. Age of onset of psychosis in siblings. Submitted for publication.
23. Hare, E.H., Price, J.S., & Slater, E. Mental disorder and season of birth; A national sample compared to the general population. *British Journal of Psychiatry*, 1974, *124*, 81–86.
24. Hare, E.H. & Walter, S.D. Seasonal variation in admissions of psychiatric patients and its relation to seasonal variation in their birth. *Journal of Epidemiological Community Health*, 1978, *32*, 47–52.
25. Watson, C.G., Kucala, T., Tilleskjor, C., & Jacobs, L. Schizophrenic birth seasonality in relation to the incidence of infectious diseases and temperature extremes. *Archives of General Psychiatry*, 1984, *41*, 85–90.

26. Torrey, E.F., Torrey, B.B. & Petersen, M.R. Seasonality of schizophrenic births in the United States. *Archives of General Psychiatry*, 1977, *34*, 1065–1070.

27. Kinney, D.K. & Jacobsen, B. Environmental factors in schizophrenia: New adoption study evidence. In L.C. Wynne, R.L. Cromwell, & S. Matthysse (Eds.) *The nature of schizophrenia*. New York: Wiley, 1978.

28. Flor-Henry, P. Psychosis and temporal lobe epilepsy: A controlled investigation. *Epilepsia*, 1969, *10*, 363–395.

29. Brown, R., Colter, N., Corsellis, J.A.N., Crow, T.J., Frith, C.D., Jagoe, R., Johstone, E.C., & Marsh, L. Post-mortem evidence for structural brain changes in schizophrenia. *Archives of General Psychiatry*, 1986, *43*, 36–42.

30. Reynolds, G.P. Increased concentrations and lateral asymmetry of amygdala dopamine in schizophrenia. *Nature*, 1983, *305*, 527–529.

31. Boklage, C.E. Schizophrenia, brain asymmetry development and twinning: Cellular relationship with etiological and possibly prognostic implications. *Biological Psychiatry*, 1977, *12*, 19–35.

32. Annett, M. *A single gene explanation of right and left handedness and brainedness*. Coventry: Lancaster Polytechnic, 1978.

33. Galaburda, A.M., Le May, M., Kemper, T.L., & Geschwind, N. Right-left asymmetries in the brain. *Science*, 1978, *199*, 852–856.

34. Crow, T.J. A re-evaluation of the viral hypothesis: Is psychosis the result of retroviral integration at a site close to the cerebral dominance gene? *British Journal of Psychiatry*, 1984, *145*, 243–253.

35. Taylor, P.J., Dalton, R., Fleminger, J.J., & Lishman, W.A. Differences between two studies of hand preference in psychiatric patients. *British Journal of Psychiatry*, 1982, *140*, 166–173.

36. Luchins, D., Weinberger, D., & Wyatt, R.J. Anomalous lateralisation associated with a milder form of schizophrenia. *American Journal of Psychiatry*, 1979, *136*, 1598–1599.

37. Luchins, D., Pollin, W., & Wyatt, R.J. Laterality in monozygotic schizophrenic twins: An alternative hypothesis. *Biological Psychiatry*, 1980, *15*, 87–93.

38. Kendall, R.E., & Gourlay, J. The clinical distinction between the affective psychoses and schizophrenia. *British Journal of Psychiatry*, 1970, *117*, 261–266.

39. Lishman, W.A., & McMeekan, E.R.L. Hand preference patterns

in psychiatric patients. *British Journal of Psychiatry*, 1976, *129*, 158–166.

40. Sackheim, H.A. Decina, P. Lateralised neuropsychological abnoemalities in bipolar adults and in children of bipolar probands. In P. Flor-Henry & J. Gruzelier (Eds.), *Laterality and Psychopathology*. Amsterdam, Elsevier, 1983.

41. Andreasen, N.C., & Powers, P.S. Creativity and psychosis. *Archives of General Psychiatry*, 1975, *32*, 70–73.

42. Jamison, K.R. In F.K. Goodwin & K.R. Jamison (Eds.), *Manic-depressive illness*. Oxford University Press, 1985.

43. Karlsson, J.L. Genetic association of giftedness and creativity with schizophrenia. *Hereditas*, 1970, *66*, 171–181.

44. Paquin, C.E. & Williamson, V.M. Temperature effects on the rate of Ty transposition. *Science*, 1984, *226*, 53–55.

45. Hickey, D.A. Selfish DNA: A sexually-transmitted nuclear parasite. *Genetics*, 1982, *101*, 519–531.

46. Kidwell, M.G. Evolution of hybrid dysgenesis determinants in Drosophila Melanogaster. *Proceedings of the National Academy of Science*, 1983, *80*, 1655–1659.

Chapter 4

A STUDY OF THE IMMUNOLOGICAL STATE OF SCHIZOPHRENIC PATIENTS

Stavroula Theodoropoulou-Vaidaki, M.D.
Costas Alexopoulos, M.D. and
Costas N. Stefanis, M.D.

Cellular and humoral immunological abnormalities in schizophrenia have been reported as early as the beginning of this century. Nevertheless a systematic study of the immunological state of schizophrenic patients began only in the 1960s and the literature on the subject is steadily expanding. Despite the sizable number of reported papers the data published so far are mostly fragmentary and often contradictory.[1-5, 21-25] Thus a solid basis to hypothesize an immunological abnormality as a contributing factor to schizophrenia is currently lacking. Difficulty in interpreting published results is due to the small number and inhomogeneity of the patients studied, to the great variability in methodology, and to the fragmentary investigation of immunological parameters. It is for these reasons that in our present study several in vivo and in vitro immunological parameters were simultaneously investigated, paying careful attention to the selection of patients, using a control group for comparison, and keeping strict experimental conditions throughout the study.

MATERIAL AND METHODS

Patients.   A total of 15 schizophrenic patients were studied in comparison with 15 normal subjects. All patients attended the Second Unit of Psychiatry at Dromokaition Hospital, Athens. Diagnosis of schizophrenia was based on strict application of DSM III criteria.[6] Patients were eligible for the study if:

Disease duration was no longer than 60 months.

Age was less than 35 years.

They had no neuroleptic medication for at least 12 months.

No other disease was present.

The control group consisted of members of the medical and nursing staff of the hospital, who showed no evidence of any somatic or mental disease, and were not taking drugs during the study period.

Immunological parameters.   The following parameters were studied.

Skin tests to PPD, streptokinase-streptodornase (SK-SD) and candida albicans (CA) antigens.

Number of circulating lymphocytes in the peripheral blood and detailed morphology.

T and B lymphocytes number in the peripheral blood.

In vitro cultures of peripheral lymphocytes in the presence of phytohemagglutinin (PHA).

Migration inhibition test (MIF test) of peripheral mononuclear cells, using PHA as antigen.

Methodology.   The following methods were used to study the above parameters.

Skin tests.   Purified tuberculin (PPD, Institute of Pasteur, Athens) at a strength of 2 units/0.1ml, candida albicans (Bencard) in a final concentration of 0.33 percent and streptokinase-streptodornase (Varidase, Lederle) in fresh solution and a final concentration of 100 units/0.1 ml, were used as recall antigens. A small quantity of 0.1 ml was injected intradermally in the medial part of the forearm, using an insulin syringe. An equal quantity of normal saline was injected simultaneously in the opposite forearm for control purposes. Skin reaction was read 48 and 72 hours later and graded as follows: Positive (+)=induration of 5–9 mm, positive (++)=induration of 10–14 mm, positive (+++)=induration of 15–19 mm and positive (++++)=induration>20 mm. Erythema without induration was discounted.

Enumeration of peripheral blood lymphocytes.   Thirty-three milliliters of venous blood were drawn from each control subject and schizophrenic patient. Three milliliters were collected in a small plastic tube with EDTA as anticoagulant and this quantity was used for white cell enumeration, differential count estimation, and lymphocyte morphological study, using very thin cell smears. The remaining 30ml were collected in heparinized plastic tubes. This blood was used for T and B enumeration, lymphocyte cultures, and migration inhibition tests. White blood cell enumeration was performed in the coulter counter while the differential count was estimated by microscopical counting of 300 white cells for each slide.

The estimation of the morphology of lymphocytes was performed by an independent experienced hematologist, using code-numbered slides. The following three categories of lymphocytes were used:

Normal lymphocytes: mature small lymphocytes.

Atypical lymphocytes: lymphocytes of twice the normal size, with abundant basophilic cytoplasm without granules and with large nucleus and coarse chromatin. On several occasions the nucleus was indented.

Transformed lymphocytes: lymphocytes with abundant hyaline cytoplasm and large lightly stained nucleus. In some cases the nucleus appeared cloverlike.

Lymphocyte separation and T and B cell enumeration.   Lymphocytes were separated from the venous blood by differential centifugation on Ficoll/Hypaque gradient.[7] The purity and viability of mononuclear cells so obtained were more than 95 percent.

T lymphocytes enumeration was performed by E_N-rosetting test as previously described.[8] In this method neuraminidase pretreated sheep red cells were used. As E_N-rosette positive was considered any lymphocyte with four or more red cells adherent to its surface membrance.

For B lymphocytes enumeration the EAC-rosetting test was used.[9] As EAC-rosette positive was considered any lymphocyte with three or more adherent red cells.

In vitro culture of peripheral lymphocytes with PHA. Details of the method used follow:

Cultures of lymphocytes from schizophrenics were performed in pairs with normal people in order to have absolutely comparable conditions. Purified PHA (p-PHA, Wellcome) in a concentration of $1\mu g/ml$, was used as mitogen. $100\mu l$ of suspension of lymphocytes in RPMI-1640 containing 1.5×10^6 cells were mixed with equal volume of RPMI-1640, containing 10% fetal calf serum (Gibco), 200U/ml of penicillin and $100\mu g/ml$ of streptomycin, in disposable plastic plates with 96 wells and plastic cover (Nunc). Each test was set up in triplicate. Equal numbers of control wells were filled up as above, omitting only the PHA mitogen. The plate was put in a humidified atmosphere, gassed with 5% CO_2 (Gaspak, BBL) and incubated for 48 hours at 37° C.

Lymphocyte transformation was estimated by light microscopy using cytocentrifuged slides (Cytospin, Shandon Southern) and May Grünwald-Giemsa staining. The estimation was performed by the same independent hematologist, who estimated lymphocyte morphology, again using code-numbered slides.

The terminology used was as follows:

Normal lymphocytes: small mature lymphocytes.

Intermediate cells: lymphocytes larger than normal with more abundant cytoplasm, demonstrating some degree of basophilia and nucleus with coarse chromatin but without nucleoli.

Blast cells: large cells with abundant, strongly basophilic cytoplasm, nucleus with very coarse chromatin and 2 or more nucleoli.

The results of the in vitro cultures of lymphocytes with and without PHA were expressed as follows:

Estimated percentage of blast cells.
Estimated percentage of transformed cells.
Blastic transformation index (BTI).
Cumulative transformation index (CTI).
The latter two indexes are given by the following formulae:

$$BTI = \frac{Blasts\ \%\ in\ presence\ of\ PHA}{Blasts\ \%\ in\ absence\ of\ PHA}$$

$$CTI = \frac{Cumulative\ transformation\ \%\ in\ presence\ of\ PHA}{Cumulative\ transformation\ \%\ in\ absence\ of\ PHA}$$

Migration inhibition test (MIF test). The ability of peripheral lymphocytes from schizophrenics and controls to produce the lymphokine Migration Inhibitory Factor (MIF), when stimulated with PHA, was estimated in the present study using the mononuclear inhibition test as described by Ng and Alexopoulos.[10] As antigen we used purified PHA in a concentration of $0.5\mu g/ml$.

Results were expressed as Migration Index (MI) given by the following formula:

$$MI = \frac{Area\ of\ migration\ in\ presence\ of\ PHA}{Area\ of\ migration\ in\ absence\ of\ PHA}$$

Statistical methods. For statistical analysis of our results we used the t-tests of the means and the paired t-test.

RESULTS

The clinical characteristics of schizophrenic patients are shown in Table 4-1. There were 11 men and four women and the mean age was twenty-six years.[18-31] Minimal duration of disease was 6 months and maximal 60 months. No patient was on neu-

Table 4-1.   **Characteristics of the Patients**

No/Sex/Age	Type of Schizophrenia	Duration of illness (months)	Off treatment (months)
1/F/18	Disorganized	12	—*
2/M/29	Paranoid	24	12
3/M/26	Paranoid	12	—
4/M/25	Paranoid	60	12
5/M/29	Undifferentiated	60	24
6/F/24	Disorganized	60	12
7/F/28	Undifferentiated	36	36
8/M/21	Paranoid	36	12
9/F/24	Disorganized	24	—
10/M/23	Paranoid	6	—
11/M/30	Disorganized	60	24
12/M/26	Disorganized	60	12
13/M/29	Undifferentiated	6	—
14/M/25	Paranoid	12	—
15/M/31	Residual	60	36

*—: Never received neuroleptic medication

roleptic medication for the past year and six had never taken any neuroleptic medication.

Skin reactivity.   All 15 schizophrenics were PPD negative, 14 CA negative, and 12 SK-SK negative. Furthermore, 13 out of 15 (86.6%) were anergic to all three antigens used, while 14 out of 15 (93.3%) were anergic to two. Among the controls, seven were PPD negative, four SK-SD negative, and six CA negative. Only 3 out of 15 (20%) were anergic to two antigens and none to all three (Figure 4-1).

Peripheral blood lymphocytes.   The number of circulating lymphocytes and the percentage of atypical and transformed cells are shown in Table 4-2 both for the control group and schizophrenic group. No difference was found between the number of peripheral lymphocytes of schizophrenics (2377/mm³) and the mean 2317/mm³ of the controls. Nevertheless, 8.4 percent of circulating lymphocytes in schizophrenics were atypical lymphocytes while 16.3 percent demonstrated a degree of transfor-

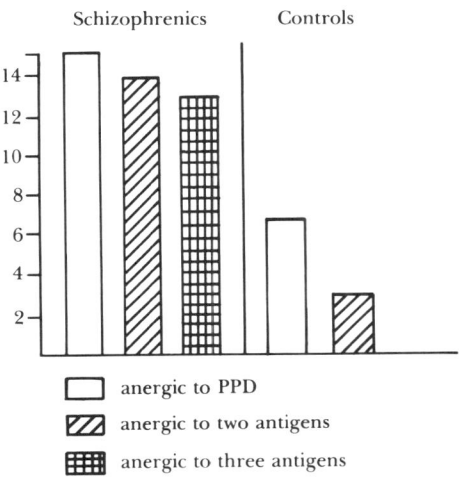

Figure 4-1. Skin reactivity to PPD, SK-SD, and CA.

mation. These figures were significantly higher ($p<0.001$) than the corresponding 2.9 percent and 4.5 percent for the controls.

B lymphocytes number. The percentage and the mean number of circulating B lymphocytes were found 23.9 percent and 581.9/mm^3 respectively in the schizophrenic patients and both values were significantly higher ($p<0.001$) than the corresponding 15 percent and 346.7/mm^3 of the controls (Table 4-3).

T lymphocytes number. The percentage of the circulating T lymphocytes was found to be 67.4 percent in schizophrenic patients and this value was significantly lower ($p<0.001$) than the corresponding 74.8 percent of the controls. On the other hand, the absolute number of circulating T lymphocytes (1606/mm^3), although lower in schizophrenics was not significantly different ($p>0.4$) from the corresponding number of 1730/mm^3 for the controls (Table 4-3).

Blastic transformation of lymphocytes. The results of a 48-hour culture of lymphocytes, under optimal conditions, with and without PHA, are shown in Tables 4-4, 4-5, and 4-6 for the schizophrenic patients and controls.

Analysis of these results demonstrated that:

The mean value of blastic transformation of unstimulated

Table 4-2.   **Lymphocytes/mm³ and Percentage of Atypical and Transformed Lymphocytes in the Peripheral Blood of Controls and Schizophrenics**

	Controls	Schizophrenics	P value
Lymphocytes/mm³	2317±526	2377±660	p>0.70
Atypical lymphocytes %	2.9±1.1	8.4±2	p<0.001
Transformed lymphocytes %	4.5±1.6	16.3±4.7	p<0.001

Table 4-3.   **Absolute Numbers and Percentages of B and T Lymphocytes in the Peripheral Blood of Schizophrenics and Controls**

	B-lymphocytes		T-lymphocytes	
	No/mm³	%	No/mm³	%
Schizophrenics	581.9±191.5	23.9±4.7	1606±466	67.4±4.9
Controls	346.7±81.2	15±2.2	1730±383	74.8±3.3
P value	p<0.001	p<0.001	p>0.40	p<0.001

lymphocytes was 39.5 percent in the schizophrenics compared with a mean of 1.16 percent for the controls, a highly significant difference (p<0.001, Table 4-4).

The mean value of the cumulative transformation of unstimulated lymphocytes was 76.5 percent for the schizophrenics compared with 43.97 percent for the controls, again a highly significant difference (p<0.001).

The mean blastic transformation index (BTI) of lymphocytes from controls was found 31.5, significantly higher (p<0.001) than the corresponding mean 1.12 of the schizophrenics.

The mean cumulative transformation index (C.T.I.) of lymphocytes from the controls was found 2.22, significantly

**Table 4-4. In Vitro Culture of Peripheral Lymphocytes
from 15 Schizophrenics and 15 Controls,
in Absence of PHA**

	No	Percentage of transformed cells	
		Blasts	Transformed
Schizophrenics	15	39.5±14.3	76.5±7.92
Controls	15	1.16±1.2	43.97±17
P value		p<0.001	p<0.001

**Table 4-5. Blastic and Cumulative Transformation
Indexes of Peripheral Lymphocytes from Controls and
Schizophrenics after Stimulation with PHA**

	Transformation indexes	
	BTI	CTI
Controls	31.5±18.3	2.22±0.71
Schizophrenics	1.12±0.35	0.98±0.12
P value	p<0.001	p<0.001

**Table 4-6. In Vitro Cultures of Peripheral
Lymphocytes from 15 Schizophrenics and 15 Controls
in Presence of PHA**

	No	Percentage of transformed cells	
		Blasts	Transformed
Schizophrenics	15	41.7±14	74.5±9.4
Controls	15	45.9±12.3	86.87±2.8
P value		p>0.30	p<0.001

higher (p<0.001) than the corresponding 0.98 from the schizophrenics (Table 5).

Finally, the mean blastic transformation of PHA stimulated lymphocytes from schizophrenic patients (41.7%) was not different from the corresponding mean of the controls (45.9%). On the contrary, the mean cumulative transformation of PHA stimulated lymphocytes of schizophrenic patients (74.5%) was significantly lower (p<0.001) than the corresponding mean 86.87 percent of controls (Table 6).

Migration inhibition test (MIF test). Migration indexes of peripheral mononuclear cells from schizophrenic patients and controls, in the presence of PHA, are given in Table 4-7. The mean migration index for the schizophrenic patients (0.72) was significantly (p<0.01) higher than the mean 0.43 for the controls.

DISCUSSION

Although immunological abnormalities in schizophrenic patients have been suggested by previous studies,[1, 2, 11-15] the differences in methodology, the small size and inhomogeneity of patient samples pose considerable difficulties in interpreting the published results. From this point of view, the careful selection of patients, the simultaneous use of controls, the simultaneous study of several in vivo and in vitro immunological parameters, and the strict experimental conditions we used in our study render our results particularly relevant.

The observed skin anergy in the vast majority of our schizophrenics, in the absence of any immunosuppressive treatment, indicates the existence of a serious defect in the cellular immunity of these patients. The existing information on skin reactivity of schizophrenic patients is scanty in the literature.[16]

The number of circulating lymphocytes was no different between schizophrenics and controls. Nevertheless, detailed morphological study of peripheral lymphocytes from schizophrenics, using very thin smears and May Grünwald-Giemsa staining, demonstrated the presence of a high percentage of transformed cells. Although some transformed lymphocytes were also found in the peripheral blood of the controls, there was a highly significant difference between the two groups.

Table 4-7. Migration Indexes of Mononuclear Cells
from the Peripheral Blood of Schizophrenics
and Controls in Presence of PHA

No	Schizophrenics	Controls
1	0.82	0.48
2	0.75	0.42
3	0.64	0.48
4	0.63	0.50
5	0.73	0.47
6	0.65	0.37
7	0.82	0.34
8	0.65	0.43
9	0.58	0.49
10	0.67	0.33
11	0.77	0.52
12	0.76	0.48
13	0.83	0.37
14	0.70	0.40
15	0.76	0.38
	$\bar{x}$ 0.72±0.08	$\bar{x}$ 0.43±0.06

These transformed lymphocytes have been also described as atypical or P-cells by others.[11, 14, 17, 18] The reasons for an increased number of atypical lymphocytes in the peripheral blood of schizophrenic patients are not known. They may indicate the presence of a miscellaneous viral infection,[18–20] an immunological response to an X antigen, or they may well be associated with antipsychotic therapy.[17] Their functional activities and their possible etiological association with schizophrenia deserve further investigation.

In our study the percentage and absolute number of B lymphocytes were significantly higher in the schizophrenics than in the controls. Increased percentage of B lymphocytes in the peripheral blood of schizophrenic patients was reported by Vartanian[2] and DeLisi.[4] However, neither of these studies offer information on the absolute number of circulating B lymphocytes. Our finding that the absolute number of B lymphocytes was also increased indicates a real increase of B lymphocytes in the peripheral blood of schizophrenic patients. The percentage of T lymphocytes, on the other hand, was found significantly lower in the schizophrenics, compared with controls. This decrease, however, is not real, and represents a complementary effect of the actual increase in the number of circulating B lymphocytes. The absolute number of circulating T lymphocytes was not different in the peripheral blood of schizophrenics compared with the controls. This latter finding is in accord with the findings of Nyland[3] who also found a normal number of T lymphocytes in the peripheral blood of schizophrenic patients. Most of the published studies on the number of circulating T lymphocytes in schizophrenics are contradictory,[1-5] while, on the other hand, many authors refer only to the percentage of circulating T lymphocytes. As our results demonstrate, a decreased percentage does not necessarily mean a diminished number of T lymphocytes.

The most interesting findings come from the 48-hour culture of peripheral lymphocytes in vitro. Blastic transformation index and cumulative transformation index, in the presence of PHA, were found significantly diminished in schizophrenic patients compared with those of the controls and these findings strongly suggest the existence of defective cellular immunity in schizophrenics. Diminished responsiveness of lymphocytes from schizophrenics to PHA has been reported by most investigators[1, 2, 21-23] while Knowles[24] has not observed such difference. Finally, Ferguson[25] reported an increased responsiveness of lymphocytes from schizophrenics to PHA stimulation.

The demonstration, in our study, of diminished blastic transformation and cumulative transformation indexes in schizophrenic patients was associated with another two equally important observations:

That peripheral lymphocytes from schizophrenics demonstrate an increased spontaneous blastic transformation, during the 48-hour culture; and

That peripheral lymphocytes from schizophrenics cultured for 48 hours, in presence of PHA, demonstrate a blastic transformation that is not different from the corresponding figure of the controls. It must be emphasized, however, that while blastic transformation of lymphocytes is directly related to their transformation capacity in presence of antigen, blastic transformation index is grossly influenced by their tendency to spontaneous transformation. The demonstrated increased tendency of lymphocytes from schizophrenics for spontaneous transformation easily explains the finding of very low blastic transformation and cumulative transformation indexes. It also helps to explain why two investigators demonstrating in fact the same phenomena, present contradictory results according to the way they treat their findings. If results are expressed as transformation indexes, then diminished responsiveness is reported,[1, 2, 22] while if results are expressed as blastic transformation capacity, then no difference between schizophrenics and controls appears.[24]

The reasons for the increased spontaneous transformation of lymphocytes of schizophrenics are not known, but various explanations have been offered:

It is due to neuroleptic therapy.[24] Neither our patients nor the patients from other studies demonstrating increased spontaneous transformation[12, 21] were under neuroleptic medication.

It is the result of stimulation of lymphocytes by an X antigen, present in the sera of schizophrenics.[12] The observed increased spontaneous transformation in our in vitro cultures, where lymphocytes had been washed extensively speaks against this view.

It is the functional expression of atypical or P-cells which demonstrate high metabolic activity even in the absence of mitogen.[22]

We believe that the presence in the peripheral blood of schizophrenics of atypical lymphocytes, their increased spontaneous transformation, and their defective responsiveness to PHA constitute in fact three different morphologicofunctional expressions of the same phenomenon. More specifically, the presence of an X antigen, either free in the sera of schizophrenics or combined with their tissues, sensitizes their mature T lymphocytes. This antigen is adhesively bound to cellular membrane receptors of T lymphocytes, which are transformed to the atypical or P-cells. Antigenic transformation does not proceed further in vivo because it is under the immunological surveillance of the body. On the other hand, in vitro no such restrictions exist and lymphocyte transformation proceeds further up to the level of T-immunoblasts. This explains very well both the increased spontaneous transformation and the low transformation indexes in presence of PHA observed in our study. In other words, the "spontaneously" stimulated T lymphocytes in the peripheral blood of schizophrenics cannot be further stimulated by PHA. The aforementioned interpretation of our findings is supported by several published observations:

Transformed lymphocytes, similar to the atypical or P-cells, have been reported in several autoimmune diseases such as systemic lupus erythematosus, myasthenia gravis, and rheumatoid arthritis.[26,27]

Separation of atypical cells from peripheral lymphocytes of schizophrenics before setting up in vitro lymphocyte cultures "corrects" the defective response to PHA and Concavalin A.[22]

Atypical lymphocytes demonstrate a high metabolic activity.[22]

Finally, our findings from the MIF test—to follow—accord with the proposed explanation.

Migration indexes of mononuclear cells from the peripheral blood of schizophrenics, in presence of PHA, were definitely abnormal in our study. This finding first suggests, that T lymphocytes of schizophrenics cannot inhibit mononuclear cell migration when stimulated with PHA. However, scrupulous analysis of the findings indicates that exactly the opposite is true. Mononuclear migration inhibition, in the presence of PHA, is satisfactory in schizophrenic patients, but migration indexes are abnormally high because there is a strong migration inhibition expressed by their lymphocytes even in the absence of PHA. This latter finding has only one explanation: Increased spontaneous transformation of lymphocytes, during the 18 hours of incubation, is associated with spontaneous production of migration inhibitory factor (MIF).

It is therefore clear that the proposed hypothesis of sensitization of peripheral T lymphocytes of schizophrenics to an X antigen adhesively bound to the cellular surface, explains satisfactorily all our present findings and most of the published observations, concerning the behavior of lymphocytes of schizophrenics to PHA and Con A. Even more importantly, it may explain much of the existing contradictory results in the literature.

It has though to be emphasized that the hypothetical X antigen does not necessarily signify an etiopathological relation with the illness. It might be due to a miscellaneous viral infection or to an autoantigen to which T lymphocytes are partially sensitized because of an existing defect in the function of suppressor T cells.

REFERENCES

1. Liedeman, R. R., Prilipko, L. L. The behavior of T lymphocytes in schizophrenia. In D. Bergsma, & A. L. Goldstein (Eds.) *Neurochemical and immunologic components in schizophrenia*. New York: Alan R. Liss, 1978.

2. Vartanian, M. E., Kolyaskina, G. I., Lozovsky, D. V., et al. Aspects of humoral and cellular immunity in schizophrenia. In D. Bergsma, A. L. Goldstein, (Eds.) *Neurochemical and immunologic components in schizophrenia*. New York: Alan R. Liss, 1978.

3. Nyland, H., Naess, A., & Lunde, H. Lymphocyte subpopulations in peripheral blood from schizophrenic patients. *Acta Psychiatrica Scandinavica* 1980, *61,* 313–318.

4. DeLisi L. E., & Wyatt, R. J. Abnormal immune regulation in schizophrenic patients. *Psychopharmacology Bulletin*, 1982, *18,* 158–163.

5. Coffey, C. E., Sullivan, J. L., & Rice, J. R. T lymphocytes in schizophrenia. *Biological Psychiatry*, 1983, *18,* 113–119.

6. American Psychiatric Association: Diagnostic and Statistical Manual of Mental Disorders. (3rd ed.) Washington DC, 1980.

7. Boyum, A. Separation of leukocytes from blood and bone marrow. *Scandinavian Journal of Clinical Laboratory Investigation* (Suppl. 97) *21*, 77–89.

8. Alexopoulos, C. Ng, R. P. Enumeration of rosette forming cells in man—A comparison of three methods. *Immunological Communications*, 1976, *5*, 87–95.

9. Alexopoulos, C., Papayannis, A., & Gardikas, C. Increased proportion in human T lymphocytes in human tonsils and appendicitis. *Acta Haematologica*, 1976, *55*, 95–98.

10. Ng, R. P., Alexopoulos, C. Mononuclear cells migration inhibition and delayed hypersensitivity in man. *Journal of Immunological Methods*, 1976, *11*, 1–6.

11. Fessel, W. J., & Hirata-Hibi, M. Abnormal leukocytes in schizophrenia. *Archives of General Psychiatry*, 1963, *9*, 601–613.

12. Liedeman, R. R., & Prilipko, L. L. The spontaneous activation of lymphocytes in schizophrenic patients in vitro revealed by a microfluorometric method. *Journal of Psychiatric Research*, 1972, *9*, 155–161.

13. Loseva, T. M. Thymus dependent lymphocytes in the spontaneous rosette-formation reaction in schizophrenia. *Journal of Neuropathology and Psychiatry*, 1977, *77*, 692–695. (in Russian with English summary)

14. Tachibana, T., Watanabe, N., Masuko, K., et al. Atypical lymphocytes and quantitative analyses of various immunological measures. *Seishim Shinkeigaku Zasshi*, 1981, *83*, 406–417.

15. Watanabe, M., Funahashi, T., Suzuki, T., et al. Antithymic antibodies in schizophrenic sera. *Biological Psychiatry*, 1982, *17*, 699–710.

16. Sisenbaev, S. K., Melkumou, G. A., & Budnevich, R. I. Tuberculin sensitivity in psychic patients. *Probleme Tuberkulosis*, 1981, *2*, 13–15. (in Russian with English summary)

17. Fieve, R. R., Blumenthal, B:, Little, B. The relationship of atypical lymphocytes, phenothiazines, and schizophrenia. *Archives of General Psychiatry*, 1966, *15*, 529–534.

18. Hirata-Hibi, M., Higashi, S., Tachibana, T., et al. Stimulated lymphocytes in schizophrenia. *Archives of General Psychiatry*, 1982, *39*, 82–87.

19. Litwins, J., & Leibowitz, S. Abnormal lymphocytes (virocytes) in virus diseases other than infectious mononucleosis. *Acta Haematologica*, 1951, *5*, 223–231.

20. Tyrell, D. A. J., Parry, R. P., Crow, T. J., et al. Possible virus in schizophrenia and some neurological disorders. *Lancet*, 1979, *1*, 839–841.

21. Mariczq, H. R., Jarvic, L. F., & Rainer, J. D. Chronic schizophrenia,

lymphocyte growth, and nailfold plexus visualization score. *Diseases of the Nervous System*, 1968, *29*, 659–667.

22. Kovalena, E. S., Bonartzev, P. D., & Prilipko, L. L. Response of lymphocytes of patients with schizophrenia to phytomitogens Concavalin A and Phytohemaglutinin. *Bulletin of Experimental Biological Medicine*, 1978, *84*, 1136–1139.

23. Fetissova, T. K. Proliferative response of lymphocytes in peripheral blood of schizophrenic patients. *Journal of Neuropathology and Psychiatry*, 1978, *78*, 867–871. (in Russian with English summary)

24. Knowles, M., Saunders, M., & McClelland, H. A. The effects of phenothiazine therapy on lymphocyte transformation in schizophrenia. *Acta Psychiatrica Scandinavica*, 1970, *46*, 64–70.

25. Ferguson, R. M., Schmidtke, J. R., & Simmons, R. L. Effects of psychoactive drugs on in vitro lymphocyte activation, in D. Bergsma, A. L. Goldstein, (Eds.), *Neurochemical and immunologic components in schizophrenia*. New York: Alan R. Liss, 1978.

26. Hirata-Hibi, M., Arimori, S., Hayashi, K., et al. Atypical lymphocytes in myasthenia Gravisand systemic lupus erythematosus. *Jahresbericht Kurashiki Zentralhospital*, 1979, *48*, 21–29.

27. Hirata-Hibi, M., Oguchi, Y., Oohara, A., et al. Abnormal lymphocytes in rheumatoid arthritis. In *Abstracts of the 14th International Congress of Rheumatology*. Bethesda, Md, International Congress of Rheumatology, 1977.

Chapter 5

GROWTH HORMONE AND PROLACTIN RESPONSES TO THE APOMORPHINE CHALLENGE

Studies in Controls and Nonmedicated Paranoid and Nonparanoid Schizophrenics

John Hatzimanolis, M.D.,
Pantelis Rinieris, M.D.,
Manolis Markianos, Ph.D.,
George Tolis, M.D., and
Costas Stefanis, M.D.

Neurophysiological, biochemical, and pharmacological data have led to the hypothesis that a dopamine disturbance may be involved in the pathogenesis of schizophrenia. In particular, a hypersensitivity of the mesolimbic, mesocortical, and nigrostriatal dopaminergic system has been suggested.[1]

Since the in vivo testing of the above hypothesis is presently unattainable, attempts have been made to evaluate the sensitivity of the tubero-infundibular dopaminergic system by means of pituitary hormone release under a dopaminomimetic challenge. In particular, assessment of growth hormone (GH) and prolactin (PRL) release in schizophrenic patients has been reported by several authors[2-14] with variable findings. In addition to differences in research protocols, one factor that may substantially contribute to discrepancies both in results and interpretations is the fact that heavily medicated patients were used in these studies.

It is for this reason that in our present study we investigated the effects of apomorphine administration, in sub-emetic doses, on the GH and PRL secretion in schizophrenic patients who had never received psychotropic medication.

METHOD

The subjects of this study were 16 male chronic (or sub-chronic, schizophrenic patients (8 paranoids and 8 nonparanoids) and 12 male mentally healthy controls.

A satisfactory matching in age between patients and controls (26.9 ± 4.4 vs 26.2 ± 4.3, years) as well as in duration of illness between paranoids and nonparanoids (2.1 ± 1.1 vs 3.5 ± 1.9, years), was obtained.

All patients met the DSMIII criteria for the diagnosis of schizophrenia and they had never received minor or major tranquilizers. Paranoids were separated from nonparanoids according to the criteria of Tsuang and Winokur.[15]

Following the admission to the hospital, patients were allowed 4 to 6 days' adaptation period, during which they received no medication. For the controls the adaptation period was about 2 hours.

The apomorphine tests were carried out in the morning after an overnight fast. Apomorphine HCl was given as an i.v. bolus of 0.375 mg and blood samples were collected at -20, 0, +20, +40, +60, +80, and +110 minutes after the injection. Serum GH and PRL levels were determined by the use of the radioimmunoassay kits of Biodata.

Analysis of variance (ANOVA) was used for the statistical evaluation of the data.

RESULTS

Basal values of GH were not statistically different when compared among groups (paranoids vs nonparanoids, and both vs controls).

A sharp rise of GH was seen at 40 minutes in all three groups. The levels obtained were not statistically different among groups (controls, 15.4±11.9 ng/ml; paranoids, 12.2±7.0 ng/ml; nonparanoids, 13.4±8.9 ng/ml; mean ± SD).

The postpeak drop of GH was such that a t½ of 20–25 minutes could be calculated and was the same for all three groups.

Both basal (controls, 10.5±4.2 ng/ml; paranoids, 8.6±5.8 ng/ml; nonparanoids, 8.2±3.0 ng/ml; mean ± SD), and nadir values (controls, 4.9±1.9 ng/ml; paranoids, 3.7±1.4 ng/ml; nonparanoids, 3.8±1.0 ng/ml; mean ± SD) following the apomorphine administration were comparable for all three groups.

DISCUSSION

In the present study, no difference in the rise of GH following administration of apomorphine hydrochloride between control subjects and either of the two groups of schizophrenic patients (paranoids and nonparanoids) was observed. This finding indicates lack of hypersensitivity of dopamine receptors at least in the tubero-infundibular system of schizophrenic patients. Similarly, supressibility of PRL was not different among the groups indicating that dopamine receptors at the pituitary lactotropes in schizophrenics are not more sensitive than in control subjects. Since apomorphine is not capable of stimulating GH release at the pituitary level, but operates at the level of the hypothalamus, the assumption is that the dopamine-dependent driving of the somatostatinergic and somatocrininergic neurons must be comparable for the schizophrenic subgroups and similar to that of the mentally healthy controls.

Our findings are at variance with those of certain authors[2, 3, 6–10, 12, 13] and in accordance with those of others.[5, 11, 14] It is to be noted, however, that our findings derive from carefully selected and strictly diagnosed patients who had never received psychotropic medication. Thus this factor possibly interfering with receptor sensitivity can safely be excluded.

REFERENCES

1. Snyder, S.H. Neurotransmitters and CNS disease-schizophrenia. *Lancet*, 1982, 970–973.
2. Ettigi, P., Nair, N.P.V., Lal. S., et al Effect of apomorphine on growth hormone and prolactin secretion in schizophrenic patients, with or without oral dyskinesia, withdrawn from chronic neuroleptic therapy. *Journal of Neurological Neuro-Surgical Psychiatry*, 1976, *39*, 870–876.
3. Rotrosen, J., Angrist, B., Gershon, S., et al Neuroendocrine effects of apomorphine: characterization of response patterns and application to schizophrenia research. *British Journal of Psychiatry*, 1979, *135*, 444–456.
4. Meltzer, H.Y., Busch, D., & Fang, V.S. Hormones, dopamine receptors and schizophrenia. *Psychoneuroendocrinology*, 1981, *6*:17–36.
5. Meltzer, H.Y., Busch, D., So, R., et al Neuroleptic-induced elevations in serum prolactin levels: Etiology and significance. In C. Baxter, & T. Melnechuk (Eds.) *Perspectives in schizophrenia research*. New York: Raven Press, 1980.
6. Cleghorn, J.M., Brown, G.M., Kaplan, R.D., et al. Growth hormone responses to graded doses of apomorphine HCl in schizophrenia. *Biological Psychiatry*, 1983, *18*, 875–885.
7. Cleghorn, J.M., Brown, G.M., Kaplan, R.D., et al Growth hormone response to apomorphine HCl in schizophrenic patients on drug holidays and at relapse. *British J. Psychiatry*, 1983, *142*, 428–488.
8. Cleghorn, J.M., Brown, G.M., Brown, P.J., et al Longitudinal instability of hormone responses in schizophrenia. *Progress in Neuro-Psychopharmacology and Biological Psychiatry*, 1983, *7*, 545–549.
9. Ferrier, N., Johnstone, E., & Crow, T. Hormonal effects of apomorphine in schizophrenia. *British Journal of Psychiatry*, 1984, *144*, 349–357.
10. Brown, W.A., & Laughren, T. Low serum prolactin and early re-

lapse following neuroleptic withdrawal. *American Journal of Psychiatry*, 1981, *138*, 237–239.

11. Gruen, P.H., Sachar, E.J., Langer, G., et al Prolactin responses to neuroleptics in normal and schizophrenic subjects. *Archives of General Psychiatry*, 1978, *35*, 108–116.

12. Rotrosen, J., Angrist, B., Clarc, C., et al Suppression of prolactin by dopamine agonists in schizophrenics and controls. *American Journal of Psychiatry*, 1978, *135*, 949–951.

13. Tamminga, C.A., Smith, R.C., Pandey, G., et al A neuroendocrine study of supersensitivity in tardive dyskinesia. *Archives General Psychiatry*, 1977, *34*, 1199–1203.

14. Smith, R.C., Tamminga, C.A., Haraszti, J, et al Effect of dopamine agonists in tardive dyskinesia. *American Journal of Psychiatry*, 1977, *134*, 763–768.

15. Tsuang, M.T., & Winokur, G. Criteria for subtyping schizophrenia. *Archives of General Psychiatry*, 1974, *31*, 43–47.

Part II

PSYCHOPATHOLOGICAL, PSYCHOPHYSIOLOGICAL, AND COGNITIVE FACTORS

Chapter 6

RELATION OF CYCLOID PSYCHOSES TO SCHIZOPHRENIC DISORDERS OF SCHIZOAFFECTIVE TYPE

Carlo Perris, M.D.

The term "cycloid psychoses" is one of the many eponyms[1] used to label psychotic disorders that do not properly fit with traditional concepts of schizophrenia and of manic-depressive illness, and which have challenged psychiatric nosologists who find it hard to comply with the Procrustean task of forcing down all nonorganic psychotic conditions in an only dichotomous classification.

Despite the fact that the concept of cycloid psychotic disorder has been introduced in the psychiatric literature early in the twentieth century, it is still poorly understood and has not yet got a place in worldwide accepted classifications of mental disorders.

The term *zykloide Psychosen* was first used by Kleist[2] to delineate some benign forms of endogenous psychoses within the larger group of the so-called degeneration psychoses, and has to be regarded as an expression of the criticism directed both against the unitary view of dementia praecox and the all-encompassing Kraepelinian conception of manic-depressive insanity. Kleist formerly comprised in the group of disorders that he labelled "cycloid" the "excited-stuporose confusion psy-

chosis" and the "hyperkinetic-akinetic motility psychosis." However, he later included in this group the "anxious ecstatic
delusional psychosis"[3] that had been thoroughly investigated by
Leonhard.[4] Leonhard, who had earlier used the term "atypical
endogenous psychoses", later[5] shifted to that of cycloid psychoses retaining in this group the three main subtypes taken into
account by Kleist. Leonard not only suggested that cycloid psychoses were to be regarded as genotypically separate from both
manic-depressive insanity and schizophrenia, on the basis of
family studies, but also emphasized the predictive value of the
concept of cycloid psychotic disorders documenting their recurrent course not followed by defect, even in the long run.

Apparently, the conceptions of Kleist and Leonhard have
had some impact in Japan where the hypotheses by Leonhard
have been integrated into and largely confirmed by genetic research by Mitsuda[6] and Kurosawa[7] and into clinical-biological
investigations by Hatotani and his coworkers.[8, 9] Japanese
authors, however, have consistently used the term "atypical
psychoses," which is somewhat more comprehensive than
that of cycloid psychosis.

In the USA the possible occurrence of atypical manic-depressive and schizophrenic syndromes was pointed out very
early by Dunton[10] who reported cases of cyclic dementia praecox, and by Kirby,[11] who described psychotic conditions mani-
festing themselves in the form of a cataleptic stupor arising
acutely in relation to a traumatic event and showing manic-depressive manifestations in the further course. However, a mile-
stone in the North American history of psychiatric nosology was
laid down by Kasanin[12] in 1933 with the introduction of the
concept of "schizoaffective psychosis." In his seminal paper,
Kasanin described an acute psychotic condition occurring in
young men and women and characterized by an admixture of
affective and schizophrenic symptoms. He also pointed out that
in the past history of his patients there was a vague history of
previous breakdowns followed by recovery. Kasanin was very
keen in emphasizing that all of his patients had made a complete recovery and that any assumption about a definite disease
process going on to deterioration and dementia was not justified by an unbiased study of his cases. Although both Kasanin
and the discussants of his paper stressed the independence of

schizoaffective psychosis from schizophrenia, the term was introduced in the 1952 classification of the American Psychiatric Association as referring to one subtype of schizophrenia. To justify this decision, the addition to Kasanin's description was made that "on prolonged observation such cases usually prove to be basically schizophrenic in nature, i.e. deteriorate." Schizoaffective psychoses have been classified as a subtype of schizophrenia also in the successive revisions of the World Health Organization International Classification of Diseases (ICD).

More recently, a reorientation seems to have occurred in the American views of the nosological position of schizoaffective psychosis. In fact, the opinion is now prevailing that it should be regarded as belonging to the group of recurrent affective disorders.[13, 14, 15] Furthermore, it seems also that the concept of schizoaffective disorder has become interchangeable with that of "good prognosis schizophrenia" and that both good prognosis schizophrenia and "remitting schizophrenia" are now regarded as variants of affective disorders.[16, 17]

The uncertainties about the correct interpretation of the terms mentioned above are expressed in the *Diagnostic and Statistical Manual of Mental Disorders* (DSMIII) where the term "schizophreniform psychotic disorder" seems to cover the concept of good prognosis schizophrenia and where this diagnosis is grouped together with those of "brief reactive psychosis," "schizoaffective disorder," and "atypical psychosis" in a residual category of "psychotic disorders not elsewhere classified"—thus adding even more to the nosological confusion.

For reasons that are difficult to disentangle in the context of this short discussion, the concept of cycloid psychosis has never been used in the American literature. However, when reference is made to European literature, it seems that the concept of cycloid psychosis is understood as interchangeable with that of schizoaffective psychosis[18, 19, 20] and is thus following the classificatory vicissitudes of this concept.

DIAGNOSTIC CRITERIA OF CYCLOID PSYCHOTIC DISORDER

Before presenting empirical evidence supporting the view that an identification of cycloid psychosis with schizoaffective disorder as currently understood is not justified, it is proper to present the diagnostic criteria that have been successively developed by our group.[21, 22] According to these criteria a cycloid psychotic disorder is defined as follows.[22]

> An acute psychotic condition, not related to the admininstration or abuse of any drug or brain injury, occuring for the first time in subjects in the age range 15 to 50 years.
>
> The condition has a sudden onset with a rapid change from a state of health to a full-blown psychotic condition within a few hours or at most a very few days.
>
> For a defined diagnosis we require the occurrence of at least four of the following symptoms: confusion of some degree (most often perplexity or puzzlement); mood incongruent delusions of any kind, most often with a persecutory content; hallucinatory experiences of any kind, often related to themes of death; an overwhelming, frightening and pervasive experience of anxiety, not bound to particular situations or circumstances; deep feelings of happiness or ecstasy, most often with a religious coloring and an experience of illumination; motility disturbances of an akinetic or hyperkinetic type which are mostly expressional; a particular concern with death; mood swings in the background, and not so pronounced and consistent as to justify a diagnosis of an affective disorder.
>
> There is no fixed symptomatological combination. On the contrary, the symptomatology may change frequently in the course of the same episode, showing very often bipolar characteristics.
>
> The disorder shows a marked tendency to recur, but each episode is followed by recovery.

Already at his descriptive level, it is manifest that our definition of cycloid psychosis does not correspond to any of the current criteria[15, 23] of schizoaffective disorder. In contrast to diagnostic criteria for schizoaffective disorders which are biased either on the affective or on the schizophrenic component,[15] the main characteristic of our criteria of cycloid psychosis is that all symptoms are jumbled together with none prevailing long enough to arise the suspect of a consistent affective or schizophrenic disorder. Symptomatological polymorphism and symptomatological changeability are, in fact, together with a very sudden onset, the most distinguishing characteristics of cycloid psychosis. In contrast, a diagnosis of schizoaffective disorder, if warranted at all, requires most often a multidimensional approach[24] in which a "course dimension" is taken into account.

It should be pointed out that our definition of cycloid psychosis differs from the descriptions given by Leonhard[5] mainly because we maintain that the expression of the disorder in the relatively pure subtypes as described by Leonhard represents more the exception than the rule. In discussing a paper presented recently in 1984 in Berlin[25] Leonhard agreed that the variability of the symptomatology both within and between episodes was the principal characteristic of cycloid psychoses.

DISTINCTION BETWEEN CYCLOID AND SCHIZOAFFECTIVE PSYCHOTIC DISORDERS

A first preliminary comparison of patients defined as cycloid according to the 1974 set of criteria by Perris[1] with patients classified as schizoaffective (unfortunately without any clear-cut report of the criteria used) has been made by Cutting et al.[26] The authors compared 73 cycloid with as many manic, depressive, and schizophrenic, and with 49 schizoaffective patients collected at the Professorial Unit of the Maudsley Hospital in London. Besides significant differences between cycloid patients and patients with clear-cut affective and schizophrenic disorders that will not be commented upon here, the authors evidenced a few differences between cycloid and schizoaffective patients as well. In particular, cycloid patients were more often female, had a slightly more loaded family history of psychiatric disorders and were different from schizoaffective in most of the clinical features comprised in our later diagnostic criteria. Cycloid patients also showed a significantly higher annual rate of new episodes and of new admissions.

A striking evidence of the clinical distinction between cycloid and schizoaffective disorders emerged from a joint British-Swedish study reported in detail.[27, 28]

In short, three series of patients were comprised in the study: a consecutive series of 134 psychotic patients (the "Netherne series"), a series of 108 meeting Kendell's study criteria for schizoaffective psychosis and a series of 119 psychotic first admissions admitted from the Camberwell catchment area in London. The diagnoses of cycloid psychosis were made by Perris who selected 10 from the Netherne series, 13 from the Camberwell first admissions and no more than 20 (18.5 percent) from the schizoaffectives. The proportion of cycloid was higher in the subgroup with a schizomanic syndrome, 8 of 32 of whom (25 percent) were selected. Since all the patients had been consistently assessed by means of the Present State Examination,[29] it has been possible to classify them according to different diagnostic criteria and to study the concordance among the patients defined according to these criteria and those diagnosed as cycloid. Results concerning concordance with different sets of criteria for schizophrenia and for affective disorders (very low and nonsignificant K:s in all instances) are reported in the original papers. Those concerning schizoaffective disorder are presented in Table 6-1.

It can be seen that K coefficients are very low and with the exception of Kasanin's original description of schizoaffective psychosis, not statistically significant. It should be obvious from these results that to regard cycloid psychosis as a synonym for schizoaffective disorder would be a mistake.

A crossvalidation of the results just summarized has been reported in 1983 by Zaudig & Vogl[30] who applied several operational definitions for schizoaffective disorder in a series of 128 psychotic patients collected in Munich. Of the 30 patients who met diagnostic criteria for schizoaffective psychosis, only 30 percent satisfied the Perris criteria for cycloid psychoses.

DIFFERENCE IN RESPONSE TO LONG-TERM LITHIUM TREATMENT

Long-term lithium treatment has proved to have a morbidity suppressive effect on patients classified as cycloid.[31, 32] In an

Table 6-1.   Cycloid Psychosis: Concordance with Schizoaffective Disorder According to Various Diagnostic Criteria in a British Series of 119 Consecutive First Admissions for a Psychotic Disorder

DIAGNOSIS (Criteria)	Cohen K
Hospital schizoaffective	−.03
Spitzer schizoaffective	+.12
Welner schizoaffective	+.29
Kasanin schizoaffective	+.43*

*p < .05

early study, it was found that cycloid patients who complied with long-term lithium treatment showed a significant reduction in number of episodes and a significant reduction in total morbidity in comparison with patients who did not comply with medication. In addition, noncompliant patients showed a successive increase in relapses and, as a consequence, in total morbidity. These earlier findings were later verified[32] in a new series. In the later study a small group of strictly defined schizoaffective patients was also taken into account. In this small group (n=15) lithium treatment did not influence either the number of relapses or the total morbidity.

A similar finding has been reported by Maj[33] who found a significant reduction in number of episodes and in total morbidity in patients fitting the diagnostic criteria of cycloid psychosis (n=15), whereas no morbidity suppressive effect was observed in patients meeting the Welner et al.[34] criteria of schizoaffective psychosis.

On the basis of these considerations we may conclude that: For almost a century, psychiatrists all over the world have had difficulties in classifying all cases of nonorganic ("endogenous") psychoses in only the two major groups of affective or schizophrenic disorders. A large number of reports concerned with a description of syndromes that did not fit either the traditional conception of schizophrenia, or the conception of manic-depressive illness, has appeared in the literature, and a long array of eponyms has been used to designate these syndromes.

Since the early 1950s the concept of schizoaffective psychosis, introduced earlier by Kasanin[12] has been comprised in internationally accepted classifications of mental disorders as a subtype of schizophrenia.

The concept of cycloid psychosis, developed in Germany early in the twentieth century, and currently used in many other countries, is not yet taken into account in the two most widely used classification systems—the ICD and the DSM.

However, cycloid psychotic disorders seem to have consistent clinical features that differentiate them from other endogenous psychoses. The concepts most akin to that of cycloid psychosis are that of "atypical psychoses" in the Japanese literature and of *bouffée délirante* of the French psychiatrists.[35]

Recently, the term cycloid psychosis has been interpreted as interchangeable with that of schizoaffective disorder, and the later has been reintepreted as a subtype of major affective psychosis.

Evidence summarized here suggests that an identification of cycloid psychosis with schizoaffective disorder is not justified from the research results so far available.

REFERENCES

1. Perris, C. A study of cycloid psychoses. *Acta Psychiatrica Scandinavica*, 1974, supplement 253.
2. Kleist, K. Über zykloide, paranoide und epileptoide Psychosen und über die Frage der Degenerationspsychosen. *Schweiz Archives of Neurological Psychiatry*, 1928, *23*, 3–37.
3. Kleist, K. Die Gliederung der neuropsychischen Erkrankungen. *Zeitschrift für Psychiatrie und Neurologie*, 1953, *125*, 526–554.
4. Leonhard, K. Das ängstlich-ekstatische syndrom aus innerer Ursache (Angst-Eingebungspsychose) und äusserer Ursache (symptomatiche Psychosen). *Allgemeine Zeitschrift für Psychiatrie*, 1939, *110*, 101–142.
5. Leonhard, K. *Aufteilung der endogenen Psychosen*. Berlin: Akademie, 1957.
6. Mitsuda, H. *Clinical genetics in psychiatry*. Tokyo: Igaku-Shein.
7. Kurosawa, R. Untersuchung der atypischen endogenen Psychosen

(periodische Psychosen). *Psychiatric Neurology & Medical Psychology*, 1961, *13*, 364–370.

8. Hatotani, N., Ishida, C., Yra, R, et al. Psychophysiological studies of atypical psychoses. *Folia Psychiatrica et Neurologica Japonica*, 1962, *16*, 248–292.

9. Hatotani, N., Nomura, J. Neurobiology of periodic psychoses. Tokyo: Igaku-Shein, 1938.

10. Dunton, W.R. The cyclic forms of dementia praecox. *American Journal of Insanity*, 1910, *66*, 465–476; *67*, 257–278.

11. Kirby, G.H. The catatonic syndrome and its relation to manic-depressive insanity. *Journal of Mental and Nervous Disease*, 1913, *40*, 694–704.

12. Kasanin, J. The acute schizoaffective psychoses. *American Journal of Psychiatry*, 1933, *13*, 97–126.

13. Clayton, R.J., Rodin, L., & Winokur, G. Family history studies: Schizoaffective disorder, clinical and genetic factors. *Comprehensive Psychiatry*, 1968, *9*, 31–49.

14. Pope, H.G., Lipinski, J.F., Cohen, B.M., & Axelrod, D.T. Schizoaffective disorder: An invalid diagnosis? *American Journal of Psychiatry*, 1980, *137*, 921–927.

15. Maj, M. Evolution of the American concept of schizoaffective psychosis. *Neuropsychobiology*, 1984, *11*, 7–13.

16. McCabe, M.S., Fowler, J.S., Cadoret, R.J., et al. Familial differences in schizophrenics with good and poor prognosis. *Psychological Medicine*, 1971, *1*, 326–332.

17. Fowler, R.C. Remitting schizophrenia as a variant of affective disorder. *Schizophrenia Bulletin*, 1978, *4*, 68–76.

18. Procci, W.R. Schizoaffective psychosis: Fact or fiction? *Archives of General Psychiatry*, 1976, *33*, 1167–1178.

19. Tsuang, M.T. Schizoaffective disorder. *Archives of General Psychiatry*, 1979, *36*, 633–634.

20. Grossman, L.S., Harrow, M., Lechert Fudala, J., & Melzter, H.Y. The longitudinal course of schizoaffective disorders. *Journal of Nervous & Mental Disease*, 1984, *172*, 140–149.

21. Perris, C., & Brockington, I.F. Cycloid psychoses and their relation to the major psychoses. In C. Perris, C. Struwe, & B. Jansson (Eds.) *Biological Psychiatry Today*. Amsterdam: Elsevier/North Holland Biomedical Press, 1981.

22. Perris, C. Clinical prediction of outcome of psychotic conditions.

Paper presented at the WHO International Conference on Diagnosis and Classification of Mental Disorders and Alcohol- and Drug-related Problems. Copenhagen, April 13–17, 1982. In press in the Proceedings.

23. Maj, M. The evolution of some European diagnostic concepts relevant to the category of schizoaffective psychoses. *Psychopathology*, 1984, *17*, 158–167.

24. Maj, M., & Perris, C. An approach to the diagnosis and the classification of schizoaffective disorders for research purposes. *Acta Psychiatrica Scandinavica*, 1985.

25. Perris, C. Über Zykloide Psychosen und deren Stellung im Rahmen der Klassifikation endogener Psychosen. Paper presented at the Symposium on *Zur Klassifikation endogener Psychosen,* East Berlin, March 21, 1984. In press.

26. Cutting, J.C., Clare, A.W., & Mann, A.H. Cycloid psychosis: An investigation of the diagnostic concept. *Psychological Medicine,* 1978, *8,* 637–648.

27. Brockington, I.F., Perris, C., Kendell, R.E., Hillier, V.E., & Wainwright, S. The course and outcome of cycloid psychoses. *Psychological Medicine*, 1982, *12*, 97–106.

28. Brockington, I.F., Perris, C., & Meltzer, H.Y. Cycloid psychosis: Diagnosis and heuristic value. Paper presented at the Symposium on the Diagnosis and Treatment of Atypical Psychoses, Baltimore, MD, November 6–7, 1981. *Journal of Nervous & Mental Disease*, 1982, *170*, 651–656.

29. Wing, J.K., Cooper, J.E., & Sartorius, N. *Measurement and classification of psychiatric symptoms*. London: Cambridge University Press, 1974.

30. Zaudig, M., & Vogl G. Zur Frage der operationalisierung Diagnostik schizoaffektiver und zykloider Psychosen. *Archiv für Psychiatrie und Nervenkrankheiten*, 1983, *233*, 385–396.

31. Perris, C. Morbidity suppressive effect of lithium carbonate in cycloid psychosis. *Archives of General Psychiatry*, 1978, *35*, 328–331.

32. Perris, C., & Smigan, L. The use of lithium in the long-term morbidity suppressive treatment of cycloid and schizoaffective psychoses. In *Psychiatry: The State of the Art* (Vol. 3) *Pharmacopsychiatry*. New York: Plenum, 1984.

33. Maj, M. Effectiveness of lithium prophylaxis in schizoaffective psychoses: Application of a polydiagnostic approach. *Acta Psychiatrica Scandinavica*, 1984, *70*, 228–234.

34. Welner, A., Croughan, J.L., & Robins, E. The group of schizoaffective and related psychoses. *Archives of General Psychiatry*, 1974, *31*, 628–631.
35. Johnson-Sabine, E.C., Mann, A.H., Jacoby, R.J., Wood, K.H., Peron-Magnan, P., Olie, J.P. & Deniker, P. Bouffée délirante: An examination of its current status. *Psychological Medicine*, 1983, *13*, 771–778.

Chapter 7

OBSERVATIONS ON THE SCHIZOPHRENIC LANGUAGE

Marios Markidis, M.D.,
Gregory Vaslamatzis, M.D.,
Vassilis Kontaxakis, M.D., and
Urania Machera, M.D.

The curious distortions of the language of the schizophrenic patients have traditionally attracted the attention of psychopathologists as an approach to the study of schizophrenic thinking, since language was simply considered as the "expression of human thought."[1, 2] The dissociated thought processes were the basic schizophrenic symptom, according to Bleuler.[3] Language "reflects" the weakness and disconnection of the associations. The thinking disorders are also the starting point of Von Domarus,[4] as specific disturbances of syllogistic structure. "Men die—Grass dies—Men are grass." Goldstein[5, 6] observed that in both organic patients and in schizophrenics there is a reduction of capacity in abstract thinking, as a result of which the patient lives in a world of concrete reality. This "concreteness" is reflected in the language of schizophrenics, where there is an absence of words signifying categories or classes and where the words used appear as part of an object or a situation, not as a representative of it. One of Goldstein's patients used to say "kiss" instead of "mouth;" another of Storch's[7] experienced concretely the opening and the closing of doors, exclaiming: "There the doors are going to eat me up." Kasanin[8] and Benjamin[9] confirm the view of Goldstein, the latter pointing out the "literalness" of schizophrenic thinking as revealed in the interpretation of proverbs.

As to the linguistic disturbances themselves, schizophrenic language, according to Bleuler,[3] has a strong tendency to symbolism, while it has erroneously been taken as symbolic according to Goldstein,[6] since symbolism belongs to higher forms of thought which are usually impaired in schizophrenia. Arieti[10] believes that the schizophrenic loses the use of social symbols and his language is extremely rich in "paleosymbols," which are created by the individual when he selects a part or a predicate to represent the objects he wants to symbolize.

Many authors dealing with the problem of schizophrenic language tend to look simply *through* language in the way one uses mediation without paying much attention to its influence on the mediated message.[11] But "the medium *is* the message," said McLuhan.[12] They systematic linguistic study, from De Saussure to Chomsky, revealed that language is not only a mirror of the thought[2] but also the "ground" of the thought, or, as Lacan[13] put it, "the world of words creates the world of things." In connection with this creativity of the language, Jakobson,[14, 15] summarizing the work accomplished over half a century of linguistics, considers the linguistic system to be always a dual process, in which the opposed yet cooperating aspects are *code* and sociocultural *context*. The code is composed of signs that have to be put into contiguous relations according to the laws of the grammar of a given language. Naming practices follow two patterns: Metonymy allows naming through the use of contiguity. Metaphor establishes similarity either in meaning or simply in sound. Metonymy dominates scientific discourse. Metaphor dominates poetry, by expanding the discourse into figurative similarities. This dual stylistic patterning, Jakobson suggested, may be represented in all mental activity. It should also be noted that Lacan assimilates the metonymic and metaphoric processes of language to displacement and condensation respectively, that is to the two psychoanalytic mechanisms that characterize the working of the Unconscious.

In order to apply this linguistic approach to the schizophrenic disorder, it may be useful to take as a particular example a patient who has formulated a personal theory for the creation of the world, its morals and culture, wishing to base on it the changing of the world. Figure 7-1 contains the fundamentals of his philosophical system, reproduced from the patient's own manuscript and by his own permission.

This patient, like the presocratic philosophers, looks for the "first principles," in order to build on them a monistic and holistic universe, a "Persontotalmanalwayseverywhereuniversaldomination," which reproduces in a single word the processing in the metonymic axe of the language. These "principles" are hidden in the word, or rather in the letter itself. Note that composite terms like "totalmansensoemotion," etc. do not normally appear in the Greek linguistic context. The passage shown in Figure 7-2 indicates in which way the language creates the patient's world, through the arrangement of the sounds in the word *Patris* (Fatherland) and their gliding along the axis of vocal similarity.

We observe as well that the sound r, as a liquid consonant, produces the metaphor *sea* (the liquid element), which as a word does not contain this particular sound.

The dominance of the metaphoric selection, determined by the sense and more often by the vocal similarity, is clearly shown in the passage in Figure 7-3, with its anagrams and its plays upon words.

Noah is finally identified as number *One*, that is, the first man on Earth; Jesus Christ derives from *Amen*, law leads to division and unequality, and the Virgin Mary turns into the Universe bound by the Gordian knot, like a donkey to a tree. These metaphoric foundations produce the grammatically correct sentences given in Figure 7-4, where "the resurrection of the dead" will take place because, as the patient has elsewhere explained, he is the son of Anastasia, a Greek name etymologically akin to the word *resurrection*. The strange compounds "dissolutionreunion," "wholelifer," and "eachother" reveal the holistic view of the patient, to whom no division is permitted;

Figure 7-1.

GOD
(/Θeos/)

RELIGION
(/Θriskia/)

/Θarros/ courage

/eneryia/ energy

/oryanosi/ organization

/sperma/ sperm

Θ—

r—

i—

s—

k—

i—

a—

/ropes/ (tendencies)
/robot/ (robot)
/iΘiki/ (morals)
/sinoloanΘropoesΘimosinesΘima/ (totalmansensoemotion)
/kratos/ (state)
/ideodi/ (ideals)
/atomosinoloanΘropopantotepantupantokratoria/ (Persontotalmanalwayseverywhereuniversaldomination)
WAY
/oloanΘropinoyrammatariΘmoyrafomilia/ (Totalhumanletternumberwrittendiscourse)

/elefΘeria/ (freedom)
/ipotayi/ (submission)
/allayi/ (change)
/anΘropozoopsariofitofika/ (organization of mananimalfishplantseeweed)
/allayi/ (change)

Figure 7-2.

		/patris/ (Fatherland)	
p	——	/**p**ateras/	(father)
a	——	/miter**a**/	(mother)
t	——	/s**t**eria/	(land)
r	——	/Θalassa/	(sea) iγro (liquid)
i	——	/atmosfera/	(atmosphere) aerio (air)
s	——	/**s**pori/	(sperms)

the life is the whole, and each one is assimilated to the others.

In general, one finds oneself confronting a disintegration of the common linguistic code, where each unit is related metaphorically to another. Goldstein[5] believed that one would incorrectly suggest a metaphoric language in schizophrenia, where there is only "concrete realism." Nevertheless, it is precisely in the schizophrenic utterance that Bateson and his colleagues,[16] discussing von Domarus, find a "richness" in metaphor. The "paleosymbols" proposed by Arieti[10] can also hardly be conceived as anything else than metaphors. The "unpredictability" (low redundancy) of the schizophrenic speech, found on a communications's theory basis by Salzinger et al.[17] and supported by the work of Lawson et al.,[18] is probably close to an overabundance of metaphoric associations, resulting in the abnormal processing of the language. Finally, the tendency of the schizophrenic language to be disrupted by irrelevant associations[19] may be also interpreted on the same lines of metaphor via the relations of similarity, where the "irrelevant associations" are nothing more than extended meanings and assonances of the words existing in the continuity of the speech.

The overabundance of the metaphors, neglectful of the

Figure 7-3.

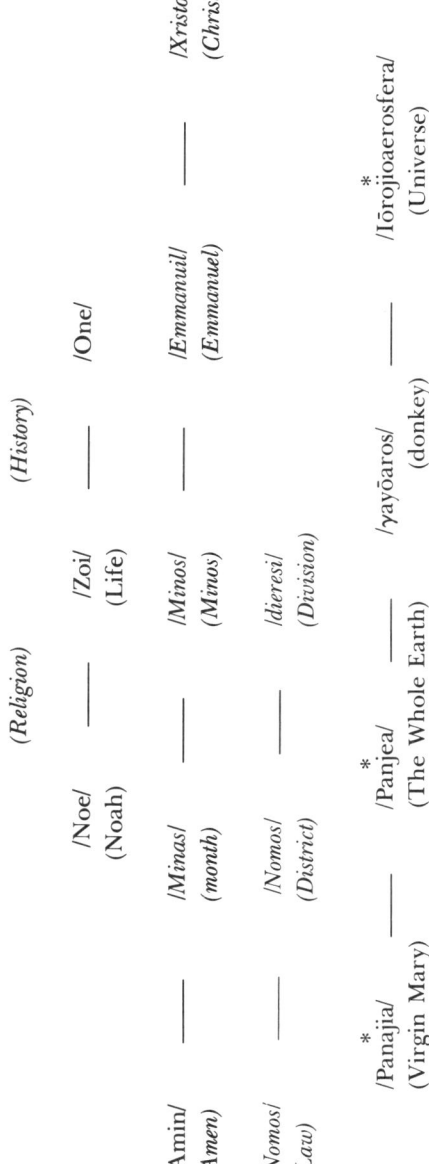

/Amin/   /Minas/   /Noe/   /Θriskia/   /Zoi/   /Istoria/   /One/   /Emmanuil/   /Xristos/
(Amen)   (month)   (Noah)   (Religion)   (Life)   (History)   —   (Emmanuel)   (Christ)

/Nomos/   /Nomos/   —   —   /Minos/   —   —   —
(Law)   (District)   (Minos)

/dieresi/
(Division)

*/Panajia/   */Panjea/   /γαγδaros/   —   */Ιōrojioaerosfera/
(Virgin Mary)   (The Whole Earth)   (donkey)   (Universe)

The universe (humanity) is bound by the Gordian knot (/rordios desmos/)

(*) j= γ + e or i

Figure 7-4.

I

We shall sweep away the bones of the dead, we shall accomplish the Resurrection of the dead.

II

We shall make the dissolutionreunion of the persontotalmanalway-severywhereuniversaldomination.

III

Oblivion then to the sinful past, and let's become wholelifers and eachothers.

common symbolic context of the language, is the main problem of the above presented discourse. The patient plays with words, as is normal in everyday life, but the assimilations, comparisons, and operations which he effects are usually strictly private, unrelated to the symbolic code accessible to all. Although the language is always a symbolic system in itself, this patient practically fails to utilize it as such.

As the purpose of this chapter is rather to describe than to explain this phenomenon, it does not address the question why it happens so in schizophrenia.

REFERENCES

1. Lewis, N.D.C. Preface. In J.S. Kasanin, (Ed.) *Language and thought in schizophrenia*, New York: Norton, 1964.
2. Critchley, M. The neurology of psychotic speech. *British Journal of Psychiatry*, 1964, *110*, 353–364.
3. Bleuler, E. *Dementia Praecox or the group of schizophrenias*. New York: International University Press, 1950.
4. Von Domarus, E. The specific laws of logic in schizophrenia. In J.S. Kasanin, (Ed.) *Language and thought in schizophrenia*, New York: Norton, 1964.

5. Goldstein, K. The significance of psychological research in schizophrenia. *Journal of Nervous and Mental Diseases*. 1943, *97*, 3–11.
6. Goldstein, K. Concerning the concreteness in schizophrenia. *Journal of Abnormal Psychology*, 1959, *59*, 146–148.
7. Storch, A. The primitive archaic forms of inner experiences and thought in schizophrenia. *Journal of Nervous and Mental Diseases, Monograph Series*, 1924, *36*.
8. Kasanin, J.S. The disturbance of conceptual thinking in schizophrenia. In J.S. Kasanin (Ed.) *Language and thought in schizophrenia*. New York: Norton, 1964.
9. Benjamin, J.D. A method for distinguishing and evaluating formal thinking disorders in schizophrenia. In J.S. Kasanin (Ed.) *Language and thought in schizophrenia*. New York: Norton, 1964.
10. Arieti, S. Some aspects of language in schizophrenia. In Heinz Werner (Ed.) *On Expressive Language*. Papers presented at the Clark University Conference on Expressive Language Behavior. Worcester, Mass., Clark University Press, 1955.
11. Shands, H.C. & Meltzer, J.D. *Language and psychiatry*. The Hague-Paris: Mouton, 1973.
12. McLuhan, M. *Understanding media*. New York: McGraw-Hill, 1965.
13. Lacan, J. The agency of the letter in the unconscious or reason since Freud. In *Ecrits—A selection*. London: Tavistock, 1977.
14. Jakobson, R. Two aspects of language and two types of aphasia disturbances. In R. Jakobson & M. Halle (Eds.) *Fundamentals of language*. La Haye, 1956.
15. Jakobson, R. *Essais de linguistique générale*. Paris: Les Éditions de Minuit, 1963.
16. Bateson, G., Jackson, D.D., Haley J., & Weakland, J. Toward a theory of schizophrenia. *Behavioral Science*, 1956, *1*, 251–264.
17. Salzinger, K., Portnoy, S., & Feldman, R. Verbal behavior in schizophrenics and some comments toward a theory of schizophrenia. Cited in B. Maher, The language of schizophrenia. *British Journal of Psychiatry*, 1972, *120*, 3–17.
18. Lawson, J.S., McGhie, A., & Chapman, J. Perception of speech in schizophrenia. *British Journal of Psychiatry*, 1964, *110*, 375–380.
19. Pavy, D. Verbal behavior in schizophrenia: a review of recent studies. *Psychological Bulletin*, 1968, *70*, 164–178.

Chapter 8

COGNITIVE PERFORMANCE IN SCHIZOPHRENIA AND ITS RELATION TO TREATMENT, PSYCHOPATHOLOGY, AROUSAL, AND ANXIETY

Aris Liakos, M.D.,
Stavroula Yannitsi, M.D., and
Sotiris Loukas, Ph.D.

It has long been accepted that cognitive performance is impaired in schizophrenia.[1] Various explanations have been proposed for this phenomenon, based on theories of impaired information processing, supposed to be specific to schizophrenia. Broadbent[2] suggested a model of impairment of selective attention, "sensory filter" defect, or "pigeonholing" which has to do with the priority of incoming stimuli.[3] Other investigators explain the disorder by a theory of a malfunctioning response filter[4] or defective "allocation policy"[5] which emphasizes extensive attention to inappropriate stimuli.

Irrespectively, however, of the theoretical explanations of performance deficit specific to schizophrenia, performance in general is know to depend on the arousal level and on anxiety. The relationship takes the form of an inverted U, with optional performance occurring at moderate levels of arousal, and poor performance at both extremes.[6, 7]

Furthermore, a number of studies show that the level of arousal is disturbed in schizophrenia. Some older reports conclude that arousal in schizophrenia is abnormally low,[8] and others that it is abnormally high.[9, 10] Ax and colleagues[11] conclude that a substantial variability in arousal levels exists in schizophrenia, the majority of patients falling in the low or high extreme of the range. It has been additionally suggested that schizophrenics may vary from states of under- or overarousal at different times.[12] McGhie[13] also added that schizophrenics suffer from both high and low levels of arousal, depending on the arousal component considered.

It is therefore reasonable to suppose that the performance deficit in schizophrenia is also due to the arousal level disturbances. The present investigation has been designed to test this hypothesis. A significant confounding factor in research with schizophrenics is drug therapy. Most schizophrenics are under tranquilizers which affect arousal level. It also affects psychopathology which is evidently related to performance. We have therefore designed the experiment to take account of these factors.

METHODS

Subjects.

Drug-free schizophrenic patients, admitted to Eginition University Clinic over a period of 2 years, were used as material for the study. All drug-free schizophrenic admissions were initially considered. If they were free of medication for a period of at least 2 weeks they were examined by two experienced psychiatrists, who interviewed the patients and examined their case records. The patients who met the DSM III diagnostic criteria for schizophrenia were included in the study. A total of 38 admissions were drug free on admission during the above named period. Six of these did not meet DSM III criteria. Four were very disturbed and the staff used medication before they could be included in the study. Three did not give their consent for the experiment. Another five patients were unable to cooperate with performance procedure and were excluded. The remaining 20, 13 male and 7 female, were included in the study. Their mean age was 26.3 (±7.6). Diagnostic categories according to DSM III criteria were the following: 6 undifferentiated, 4 disorganized, 2 residual, and 8 paranoid.

Psychometric Tests Used.

Psychopathology was measured with the Brief Psychiatric Rating Scale (BPRS),[14] and anxiety with Spielberger's State-Trait Anxiety Inventory (STAI).[15] Both instruments have been translated and validated in Greece.

Procedure.

At 10 a.m. of day of testing patients completed the STAI. They were then seen for completion of the BPRS and at 3 p.m. they were tested in the laboratory for performance and arousal level. Patients were subsequently submitted to a standard regime of chlorpromazine treatment (300mg daily) for a period of 2 weeks. At the end of treatment period the same procedure (except for the DSM III assessment) was repeated.

Laboratory Tests.

Performance was measured with the delayed auditory feedback technique; this technique can be used with subjects of all intellectual levels and although simple, it is quite sensitive.[16] It has also been shown that schizophrenics react to the test in the same way as normals.[17, 18] An addition task was performed under delayed auditory feedback conditions which lasted 90 seconds. Subjects were directed to add 3 to an initial number (3, 2, or 7) until directed to stop. A Lafayette 15016 instrument was used. Speed was 3/4 ips and the delay period was 0.28 sec. The final sum reached after 90 seconds, divided by the number of errors plus one was the performance score. Skin conductance level was recorded with a Lafayette 76406 instrument. A basal measurement, taken after 6 minutes of test and before DAF performance task, was used as a measure of arousal level.

Statistical Analysis.

A series of multiple regression analyses using covariance models were performed for the analysis of the experimental data. The technique used is described in detail by Cohen.[19] Performance was the dependent variable while both quantitative (psychopathology arousal and anxiety) and qualitative (subjects and treatment) variables consisted the independent variables of the regression models.

When testing groups of subjects, the wide variability between subjects accounts usually for a large proportion of variance of the measurements. We have therefore decided to control this factor. In all analyses, effects of the intersubject variance were accounted for, prior to investigating other relationships. This was achieved by including subjects into the regression by the use of dummy variables before inclusion of other variables. In this way relationship effects of drug therapy (also a dummy variable), psychopathology, arousal and anxiety (state or trait) on performance could be examined free of intersubject differences. Interaction and curvilinear relationship effects of the independent variables on performance was also considered. The F tests of significance on the individual variables were carried out as described in detail by Cohen.[19] Residual analyses showed no departures from the model assumptions of normality and constant variance.

RESULTS

A data summary is shown in Table 8-1. After treatment with chlorpromazine, there is a significant improvement in performance, reduction of psychopathology, and reduction of arousal level. Anxiety state was also significantly reduced, while anxiety trait showed no significant change. Tables 8-2, 8-3, and 8-4 show the significant relationships of performance to other variables. Drug therapy, psychopathology, and arousal, when considered separately, and after accounting for the intersubject variance, significantly affect performance. Anxiety (state or trait) has no significant effects.

Table 8-1. The Experimental Data (N = 20)

	Before Treatment		After Treatment		Paired t-test	P
	Mean	(S.D.)	Mean	(S.D.)		
PERFORMANCE	80.54	(45.90)	104.71	(49.05)	3.65	<.01
BPRS SCORE	50.55	(7.19)	44.05	(9.17)	-3.95	<.01
SCL	25.07	(16.66)	18.16	(13.00)	-2.68	<.01
A-STATE	47.65	(12.90)	41.05	(13.92)	-2.45	<.05
A-TRAIT	49.25	(13.68)	47.05	(13.64)	-1.08	n.s.

Table 8-2. The Relationship of Performance to Treatment

Independent Variables	Overall Regression				Due to the Entered Independent Variable			
	R^2	F	D.F.	P	R^2 Increment	F	D.F.	P
Subjects (19)*	.845	5.748	19/20	<.01	—	—	—	—
Drug	.909	9.486	20/19	<.01	.063	27.1	1/19	<.01

*Subjects were entered into the regression one by one. Figures in tables show the cumulative amounts, after insertion of the subjects (20) by the use of 19 dummy variables.

Table 8-3. The Relationship of Performance to Psychopathology

Independent Variables	Overall Regression				Due to the Entered Independent Variable			
	R^2	F	D.F.	P	R^2 Increment	F	D.F.	P
Subjects (19)*	.845	5.748	19/20	<.01	—	—	—	—
BPRS	.875	6.676	20/19	<.01	.030	4.605	1/19	<.05

Table 8-4. The Relationship of Performance to the Level of Arousal

Independent Variables	Overall Regression				Due to the Entered Independent Variable			
	R^2	F	D.F.	P	R^2 Increment	F	D.F.	P
Subjects (19)*	.845	5.748	19/20	<.01	—	—	—	—
SCL	.883	7.185	20/19	<.01	.038	6.182	1/19	<.05

Note that significant regression models were only those that included the variables accounting for the intersubject effects. The best of the regression models considered is given in Table 8-5. As seen in this table, psychopathology and arousal do not affect performance significantly after drug therapy is included in the model. This suggests that the treatment effect is the most important.

DISCUSSION

The above-mentioned relationships, although statistically significant, account for small degrees of variance, and appear only after covarying out the intersubject variance which is quite substantial (84,5%). This probably explains why they have not been demonstrated by previous investigators.

The success of drugs in reducing psychopathological symptoms, particularly abnormal schizophrenic behavior, is well established, but the psychophysiological mechanisms mediating these behavioral changes are not well understood.[20] Phenothiazines reduce sweat gland activity in schizophrenics and also improve cognitive functions.[21] A number of other studies provide empirical evidence suggesting that one mechanism mediating clinical improvement produced by phenothiazines is the reduction of autonomic arousal.[22, 23, 24] In contrast to these findings a Russian paper reports that CPZ increased sweating while improving the clinical condition of catatonic schizophrenics.[25] One reason for the discrepancy in these findings could be the failure to consider pre-drug variation in sweat gland activity. Schizophrenics can be excessively high or low in psychophysiological arousal levels, and drugs may respectively decrease or increase arousal to moderate levels. Tecce and Cole,[20] after reviewing relevant reports, conclude that phenothiazines generally reduce psychophysiological activity of schizophrenics and often improve clinical behavior and performance in psychological tests.

Our findings support these conclusions. They also show that

Table 8-5. The Relationship of Performance to Treatment, Psychopathology, and the Arousal Level

Independent Variables	Overall Regression				Due to the Entered Independent Variable			
	R^2	F	D.F.	P	R^2 Increment	F	D.F.	P
Subjects (19)*	.845	5.74	19/20	<.01	—	—	—	—
Drug	.909	9.48	20/19	<.01	.063	27.1	1/19	<.01
BPRS	.909	8.52	21/18	<.01	—	—	—	n.s.
SCL	.914	8.26	22/17	<.01	—	—	—	n.s.

improvement of psychopathology is the main factor associated with chlorpromazine administration and the accompanying reduction of arousal as reflected in skin conductance level is secondary to this improvement.

REFERENCES

1. Cameron, N. Schizophrenic thinking in problem solving situations. *Journal of Mental Science*, 1939, *85*,1012–35.
2. Broadbent, D.E. *Perception and communication*. London: Pergamon, 1958.
3. Broadbent, D.E. *Decision and stress*. New York: Academic Press, 1971.
4. Deutsch, J.A., & Deutsch, D. Attention: Some theoretical considerations. *Psychological Review*, 1963, *70*, 80–90.
5. Kahneman, D. *Attention and effort*. New York: Academic Press, 1973.
6. Duffy, E. *Activation and behavior*. New York: Wiley, 1962.
7. Goodman, S.J. Visuo-motor reaction times and brain stem multiple-unit activity. *Experimental Neurology*, 1968, *22*, 367.
8. Flekkoy, K. Psychophysiological and neurophysiological aspects of schizophrenia. *Acta Psychiatrica Scandinavica*, 1975, *51*, 234–248.
9. Thayer, J. & Silber, D.E. Relationship between levels of arousal and responsiveness among schizophrenic and normal subjects. *Journal of Abnormal Psychology*, 1971, *77*, 162–173.
10. Zahn, T.P., Rosenthal, D., & Lawlor, W.G. Electrodermal and heart orienting reactions in chronic schizophrenia. *Journal of Psychiatric Research*, 1968, *6*, 117–134.
11. Ax, A.F., Beckett, P.G.S., Cohen, B.D., et al Psychophysiological patterns in chronic schizophrenia. *Recent Advances in Biological Psychiatry*, 1962, *4*, 218–233.
12. Gruzelier, J.H. & Venables, P.H. Evidence of high and low levels of psysiological arousal in schizophrenics. *Psychophysiology*, 1975, *12*, 66–73.
13. McGhie, A. Attention and perception in schizophrenia. In Maher B.A. (Ed), *Progress in experimental personality research*, (Vol. 5), New York: Academic Press, 1970.
14. Overall, J.E. & Gorham, B.R. The brief psychiatric rating scale. *Psychological Reports*, 1962, *10*, 799–812.

15. Spielberger, C.D., Gorsurch, R.L. & Lushene, R.E. *Manual for the state-trait anxiety inventory.* Palo Alto: California Consulting Psychologists Press, 1970.

16. Hughes, F.W. & Forney, R.B. Comparative effects of three antihistaminics and ethanol on mental and motor performance. *Clinical Pharmacology and Therapeutics*, 1964, *5*, 414–421.

17. Sutton, S., Roering, W.C., & Kramer, J. Delayed auditory feedback in schizophrenics and normals. *Annals of the New York Academy of Sciences*, 1963, *105*, 832–844.

18. Watson, S.J. Effect of delayed auditory feedback on process and reactive schizophrenic subjects. *Journal of Abnormal Psychology*, 1974, *83*, 609–615.

19. Cohen, J. Multiple regression as a general data-analytic system. *Psychological Bulletin*, 1968, *70*, 426–443.

20. Tecce, J.J., & Cole, J.O. Psychophysiological responses of schizophrenics to drugs. *Psychopharmacologia*, 1972, *24*, 159–200.

21. Goldstein, M.J., & Judd, L.L., Roadnick, E.H., et al: Psychophysiological effects of phenothiazine administration in acute schizophrenics as a function of premorbid status. *Journal of Psychiatric Research*, 1969, *6*, 271–287.

22. Spohn, H.E. & Woodman, F.L. Span of apprehension and arousal in schizophrenia. *Journal of Abnormal Psychology*, 1970, *75*, 113–123.

23. Spohn, H.E., Thetford, P.E., & Cancro, R. The effects of phenothiazine medication on skin conductance and heart rate in schizophrenic patients. *Journal of Nervous and Mental Disease*, 1971, *152*, 129–139.

24. Bernstein, A.S. Electrodermal base level, tonic arousal, and adaptation in chronic schizophrenics. *Journal of Abnormal Psychology*, 1967, *72*, 221–232.

25. Lynn, R. Russian theory and research on schizophrenia. *Psychological Bulletin*, 1963, *60*, 486–498.

Chapter 9

ELECTRODERMAL LATERALITY INDICES IN PARANOID SCHIZOPHRENICS

Andreas D. Rabavilas, M.D.
John A. Liappas, M.D.
Costas N. Stefanis, M.D.

The relationship between hemispheric asymmetry and bilateral electrodermal activity (EDA) has been subject to extensive research since the mid-1970s. The evidence accumulated thus far does not unquestionably relate bilateral EDA to hemispheric functioning. It has been found that EDA is controlled not only by cortical but also by brainstem exhitatory and inhibitory neural systems, a fact leading to equivocal interpretations of the relevant literature. However, most authors agree that when EDA asymmetry is clearly demonstrated, this is very likely to reflect a functional asymmetry of the cerebral hemispheres.[1] In this context, bilateral EDA recordings appear to provide a potentially useful method for the study of psychopathological conditions, particularly those associated with some disturbance of attention. Such an approach has already been applied to the study of schizophrenia and affective disorders.[2]

With regard to schizophrenia, the current laterality theory trends, based on EEG, neuropsychological, and behavioral data, support the view that hemispheric differences in this disorder may be due to either left-sided temporolimbic dysfunction or some disturbance of transmission between hemispheres at the level of corpus callosum.[3, 4] With respect to EDA laterality differences, most of the available evidence suggests that the electrodermally responsive schizophrenic patients show predominantly higher right than left hand responses.[5-8] This has been interpreted as an additional evidence, compatible with previous laterality findings, indicating a left hemispheric dysfunction. However, such interpretation is confounded by a number of factors. These include technical factors, such as EDA assessment procedures and experimental settings, clinical factors, such as subtyping of the patients, or the course and prognosis of the illness, exogenous factors, such as drug-induced interference, and finally, neurophysiological factors, such as the probable differential lateral hemispheric influences on tonic and phasic EDA.[4]

In spite of these difficulties, EDA lateral asymmetry differences have been interestingly involved in the diagnostic process. In a previous study,[9] the relation between the direction of EDA response asymmetry to schizophrenic symptoms has been examined. Schizophrenic symptoms and signs were compared between two patient groups defined by EDA asymmetry, i.e. patients with larger right than left hand responses (R>L patients) and patients with larger left than right hand responses (L>R patients). It was found that the R>L patients exhibited predominantly "negative" symptoms, while L>R patients had mostly "positive" symptoms. These data were based on patients most of whom suffered from nuclear schizophrenia (CATEGO diagnosis) and the EDA data were confined to the stimulus elicited phasic responses.

The relevance of these two symptom groups delineated through EDA response asymmetries to what many authors have referred to as the "paranoid/nonparanoid" distinction has been put forward.[10] Furthermore, the need for separating hemispheric lateral influences on tonic and phasic EDA has also been underlined,[4] particularly in view of the reservations concerning the directional parallelism between phasic and tonic EDA lateral asymmetries.[9, 11]

The purpose of this chapter is to examine the above stated findings[9] from a different perspective by investigating (a) EDA phasic and tonic asymmetries in a group of patients with predominantly "positive" symptoms, and in particular, paranoid schizophrenics, and (b) the relation of both phasic and tonic EDA lateral differences to schizophrenic symptomatology.

METHOD

Twenty-eight dextral patients suffering from paranoid schizophrenia took part in this study. Patients were selected by means of the DSM III criteria. The demographic and clinical features of these patients are shown on Table 9-1.

Patients' symptoms were evaluated on the Brief Psychiatric Rating Scale (BPRS)[12] by two independent assessors. Interrater reliability to various BPRS items ranged from 0.87 to 0.96. Following this procedure, patients underwent the psychophysiological assessment.

EDA was recorded bilaterally between 8 and 10 a.m. on a 16103 Lafayette polygraph, with the patients sitting in comfortable chairs in the psychophysiological laboratory of the hospital. Ag/AgCl electrodes (1 inch^2 area) were applied with a slightly hypotonic electrode jelly on the distal phalanges of the first and second fingers of both hands.

Following a 5-minute rest, a series of stimuli were administered. These stimuli consisted of 15 100 dB-1000 Hz-1 sec tones presented binaurally through earphones from a Masden Tone generator, at random intervals (20–80 sec).

Skin conductance level (SCL) was sampled every min during the rest period and after 1st, 5th, 10th, and 15th tone. For each hand, the overall mean was utilized for the subsequent analysis.

Skin conductance response amplitude (RA) was defined as the first increase in skin conductance of at least 0.05 μmho occurring between 0.8 and 5 sec after stimulus onset. For each hand, the mean RA was calculated for the subsequent analysis.

A spontaneous fluctuation (SF) of skin conductance per min was calculated as the responselike increase of skin conductance of at least 0.05 μmho, which was unrelated to the 0.8-5 sec poststimulus window.

Table 9-1. Demographic and Clinical Features of the Patients

N	28
SEX (male/female)	14/14
AGE (mean/range)	30.6 yrs/21–50 yrs
EPISODE TREATED (mean/range)	1.9/1–5
DRUG FREE PERIOD (mean/range)	2.7 wks/2–4 wks
AGE OF ONSET (mean/range)	25.2 yrs/20–38 yrs
TIME SINCE FIRST EPISODE (mean/range)	5.4 yrs/1–15 yrs
LENGTH OF HOSPITALIZATION (mean/range)	14.2 mos/1 mo–5 yrs
D.S.M. III DIAGNOSIS (Type)	295.3
INCIDENCE OF SYMPTOMS (%)	
Hallucinations (persecutory–aural)	32
Delusions: Persecutory and/or jealous	75
Grandiose	28.5
Hypochondriacal	40
EDA RESPONSIVENESS (%)	100

Ratio scores were utilized as laterality indices, in which the asymmetries of the measures taken were calculated in the form (Left − Right) /(Left + Right).

Highly significant correlations between hands were found regarding the EDA measures taken in total patients (SCL = 0.965, SF = 0.926 and RA = 0.827).

RESULTS

The means and standard deviations of the EDA laterality indices used are shown in Table 9-2.

The distribution pattern of the laterality indices are presented on Figure 9-1.

It is evident that the distribution patterns of tonic EDA and phasic EDA aim at quite opposite directions. In SF and RA, most of the patients demonstrate higher left than right activity (92.8 percent and 96.4 percent of the patients, respectively). In contrast, in SCL most of the patients (78.6 percent) show higher right than left hand levels.

Table 9-2. Laterality Indices: Mean Values and
Comparison Between Sexes
(– indicates R > L, ns = nonsignificant)

	SCL	RA	SF
OVERALL MEAN	−0.023 ± 0.033	0.193 ± 0.170	0.246 ± 0.175
MALES	−0.034 ± 0.037	0.177 ± 0.203	0.222 ± 0.199
FEMALES	−0.011 ± 0.025	0.209 ± 0.134	0.270 ± 0.152
U-test	167/239	187/219	189/217
P	ns	ns	ns

The correlations of the EDA laterality indices to BPRS items are shown in Table 9-3.

In general, the trends are insignificant. SCL dextral preponderance is marginally related to "mannerisms" and RA sinistral preponderance is also marginally related to "hallucinations." SF sinistral preponderance is significantly related to "conceptual disorganization," and marginally related to "tension," "grandiosity," "suspiciousness," "hallucinations," and the total BPRS score. It should be noted that SF laterality index appears to produce more nearly significant trends as compared with the other two indices.

Between indices, SCL is negatively and significantly related to RA (−0.503, P <0.01). The remaining intercorrelations are both positive and insignificant.

The number of patients who demonstrate dextral phasic EDA preponderance is too small as to be statistically evaluated with respect to BPRS items. An attempt is therefore made to compare the six patients with tonic levels sinistral preponderance with the remaining patients on BPRS scores. It is found that R>L SCL patients show significantly more emotional withdrawal (3.9 ± 1.3 vs 1.6 ± 0.8, t= 2.60, P< 0.02), more conceptual disorganization (3.6 ± 1.5 vs 2.3 ± 0.8, t= 2.73, P< 0.02), less tension (1.4 ± 0.9 vs 2.8 ± 0.9 t= 3.10, P < 0.005), less depressive mood (1.8 ± 0.9 vs 2.8 ± 0.7, t= 2.77, P< 0.02) and more blunted affect (3.9 ± 1.3 vs 2.3 ± 1.2, t= 2.73, P< 0.02).

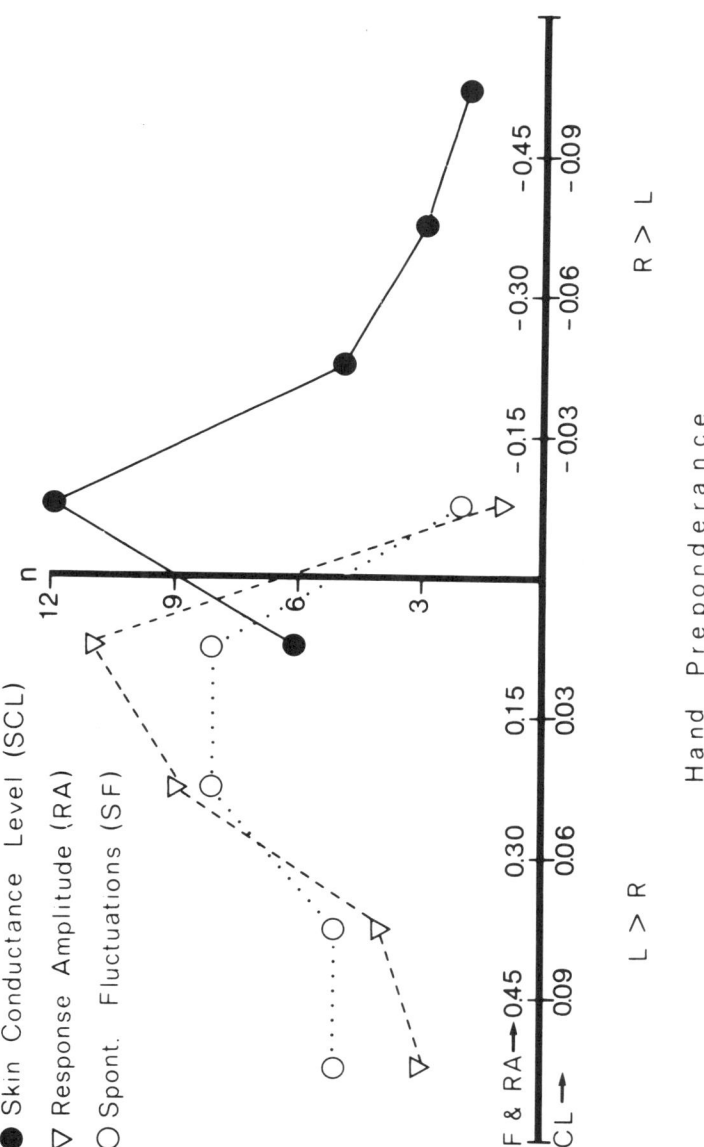

Figure 9-1. Distribution of E.D.A. laterality indices.

Table 9-3.   Correlations of EDA Laterality Indices with
BPRS Items
(* = P<0.10, ** = P<0.05)

BPRS ITEMS	SCL	RA	SF
Somatic concern	−0.128	−0.039	−0.072
Anxiety	−0.100	0.085	−0.111
Emotional withdrawal	−0.298	0.046	0.263
Conceptual disorganization	−0.104	−0.129	0.383**
Guilt feelings	−0.207	0.134	−0.096
Tension	−0.003	0.215	0.358*
Mannerisms and posturing	−0.329*	0.296	0.285
Grandiosity	−0.014	−0.092	0.334*
Depressive mood	−0.001	−0.068	−0.297
Hostility	−0.073	0.089	0.053
Suspiciousness	−0.001	−0.109	0.329*
Hallucinatory behavior	0.184	0.317*	0.302*
Motor retardation	−0.139	0.091	−0.222
Uncooperativeness	0.022	−0.220	0.050
Unusual thought content	−0.128	−0.216	0.218
Blunted affect	−0.271	0.051	0.181
TOTAL SCORE	−0.128	−0.092	0.319*

DISCUSSION

The findings of this study indicated that (a) more than 92 percent of the patients demonstrate larger left than right hand phasic EDA, (b) there is a directional opposition between lateral differences in levels and those in phasic responses and (c) the degree of EDA laterality asymmetries, with the exception perhaps of SF, is not significantly related to the severity of symptoms.

Regarding the first point, it should be remembered that the patients of this study, selected on the basis of DSM III criteria for paranoid schizophrenia, exhibit predominantly "positive" symptoms. Thus, the finding that most patients demonstrate higher left than right hand phasic EDA is consistent with the results of a previous study by Gruzelier and Manchanda.[9] Therefore, it appears that the paranoid patients of the present investigation show phasic EDA features similar to those of the "left hemisphere activation syndrome" described by the above authors. In this context, this finding corresponds with the results of other studies which reported evidence of left hemispheric activation in paranoid patients undergoing dichotic listening tasks.[13]

Regarding the second point, it is evident from the present data that tonic EDA levels are definitely higher on the right than on the left hand in 78.6 percent of the total patients. There are two alternative approaches to this finding; one could either accept the view that SCL asymmetry is labile[11] and reject this finding as being by chance, or proceed and discuss it further. In the latter case, it is interesting to note that the few patients with L>R SCL demonstrate significantly less "negative" symptoms as compared with the patients demonstrating the opposite SCL asymmetry. This may indicate that lateral asymmetry in levels could be a sensitive index of "negative" symptoms, even when these are subtle or clinically covered by the more prominent "positive" symptoms, as this might be the case regarding the patients of this study. One could go even further and support the view that a differential hemispheric influence exists in tonic and phasic EDA, in the context of the reciprocal hemispheric influences proposed by Gruzelier et al. (1981).[14] In such case, a phasic/tonic EDA laterality index could be a more appropriate measure for utilization in future research. In any case, whether this finding is related to the particular schizophrenic subgroup investigated in this study or is a finding by chance should be subject to further investigation.

Finally, regarding the last point, the severity of symptoms does not appear to be significantly related to the EDA laterality indices employed in this study. However, it should be noted that SF sinistral preponderance shows some correlational consistency of marginal significance with respect to certain symptoms as well as the total BPRS score. Since SF are widely accepted as a reliable index of general or non-specific arousal, this finding probably reflects the activation processes underlying symptom severity.

In conclusion, the results of this study support the view of a left hemispheric activation in paranoid schizophrenics. The directional opposition observed between lateral differences in levels and those in responses, as well as the relative sensitivity of SF to symptom severity, need further exploration on large samples of patients and different schizophrenic subgroups. The above findings, if confirmed, they may have a bearing on psychophysiological differentiation between symptom clusters as well as on the views concerning the hemispheric organization in psychopathological conditions.

REFERENCES

1. Hugdahl, K. Hemispheric asymmetry and bilateral electrodermal recordings: A review of the evidence. *Psychophysiology*, 1984, *21*, 371–393.

2. Flor-Henry, P. Commentary and synthesis. In J. Gruzelier, & P. Flor-Henry (Eds.) *Laterality and psychopathology*. Amsterdam: Elsevier, 1983.

3. Newlin, D.B., Carpender, B., & Golden, C.J. Hemispheric asymmetries in schizophrenia. *Biological Psychiatry*, 1981, 16, 561–582.

4. Venables, P.H. Some problems and controversies in the psychophysiological investigation of schizophrenia. In J.A. Edwards, & A. Gale (Eds.) *Physiological correlates of human behaviour*. New York: Academic Press, 1983.

5. Gruzelier, J.H. Bilateral asymmetry of skin conductance orienting activity and levels in schizophrenia. *Journal of Biological Psychology*, 1973, *1*, 21–24.

6. Gruzelier, J.H., & Venables, P.H. Bimodality and lateral asymmetry of skin conductance orienting activity in schizophrenics: Replication and evidence of lateral asymmetry in patients with depression and disorders of personality. *Biological Psychiatry*, 1974, *8*, 55–73.

7. Venables, P.H. Primary dysfunction and cortical lateralization in schizophrenia. In M. Koukkou, D. Lehmann, & J. Angst, (Eds.) *Functional states of the brain: Their determinants*. Amsterdam: Elsevier, 1980.

8. Schneider, S.J. Multiple measures of hemispheric dysfunction in schizophrenia and depression. *Psychological Medicine*, 1983, *13*, 287–297.

9. Gruzelier, J.H. & Manchanda, R. The syndrome of schizophrenia: Relations between electrodermal response, lateral asymmetries and clinical ratings. *British Journal of Psychiatry*, 1982, *141*, 488–495.

10. Gruzelier, J.H. Hemispheric imbalances as paranoid/nonparanoid syndromes. *Schizophrenia Bulletin*, 1981, 7, 662–673.

11. Gruzelier, J.H. Lateral asymmetries in electrodermal activity and psychosis. In P. Flor-Henry, & J.H. Gruzelier, (Eds.) *Hemisphere asymmetries of function in psychopathology*. Amsterdam: Elsevier, 1979.

12. Overall, J.E. & Gorham, D.R. The brief psychiatric rating scale. *Psychological Reports*, 1962, *19*, 799–812.

13. Bruder, G.E. Cerebral laterality and psychopathology : Review of dichotic listening studies. *Schizophrenia Bulletin*, 1983, *9*, 134–151.

14. Gruzelier, J.H., Eves, F.F., & Connolly, J.F. Habituation and phasic reactivity in the electrodermal system : Reciprocal hemispheric influences. *Physiological Psychology*, 1981, *9*, 313–317.

Part III

TREATMENT ISSUES

Chapter 10

DEVELOPING A GLOBAL PSYCHOTHERAPEUTIC APPROACH TO SCHIZOPHRENIA

Results of a 5-Year Follow-Up

Yrjö O. Alanen, M.D.,
Viljo Räkköläinen, M.D.,
Riitta Rasimus, M.D.,
Juhani Laakso, M.D., and
Anne Kaljonen, M.D.

We will here describe the results of an endeavor to develop a global psychotherapeutic orientation for the treatment of schizophrenia within the framework of community psychiatry, utilizing the resources of a small university hospital sharing the responsibility for the mental health services within its district.

What do we mean by "global" here? Our starting point is that the psychotherapeutic modes of treatment should be developed on the case-specific needs of the schizophrenic patients and their families. As far as we can see, the patients belonging to the schizophrenia group are heterogeneous in this respect: one patient benefits from individual therapy, another from family therapy, a third from a combination of these two; the more extensive support provided by psychotherapeutic ward community is also necessary for some of the patients, while some other patients do not need any support of this kind.

The global therapeutic orientation also includes the notion that neuroleptic medication is not an alternative to psychotherapy, but rather a support to it, and the need for medication should also be assessed separately in each case.

The starting points of our project have been shaped by goals typical of developmental work rather than research in a stricter sense. We develop the therapies taking into account the multiformity of schizophrenia, the individual needs for treatment, and the special prerequisites for successful implementation of psychotherapeutic treatments, trying simultaneously to gain some idea of the outcome of our work. Our project is carried out along the principles of action research, and it hence differs from methodologically "controlled" studies of therapeutic outcome.

NATURE AND OBJECTIVES
OF OUR THERAPEUTIC ORIENTATION

Our therapeutic orientation first came into being in 1968, when the Clinic of Psychiatry of the Turku University was founded. Together with another psychiatric hospital, the Kupittaa Hospital, and the mental health office, which is responsible for the majority of the psychiatric outpatient care, our clinic has been in charge of the psychiatric services of the mental health district consisting of the population of the town Turku (165.000, in addition to which there are, in practice, about 15.000 college and other students). This has made it possible to launch extensive efforts towards psychotherapeutically oriented treatment of schizophrenia.

Our psychotherapeutic orientation is based on the psychodynamic theory and approach. We regard schizophrenia in its most typical form as a disease based on a deep-rooted personality disorder, whose individual psychology is continuously and more or less closely related to the surrounding system of interactional relationships, particularly the dynamics of the patient's family community. It is for this reason that the therapeutic plan made for a schizophrenic patient always includes empathic and understanding exploration of both the patient himself and his family.

Both individual and family therapies have their self-evident positions in our therapeutic orientation. The third therapeutic basic dimension consists of the wards of our clinic, which are called psychotherapeutic communities.[1]

One important goal of our therapeutic orientation is to provide psychotherapeutic treatment to as many as possible of the patients for whom it is considered indicated. This presupposes a wide assortment of activities, which can be arranged by using a multiprofessional staff of therapists. Most staff members have not been given actual psychotherapeutic training, but are receiving continuous and intensive psychotherapeutic on-the-job training. Another necessary prerequisite is the development of a supervisory system of therapists.

Objectives of the Present Study

Our project covers 100 successive patients aged 16–45 years who, during the period 1976–1977, were admitted for the first time into one of the units of the community psychiatric system of the Turku district for psychosis of the schizophrenia group. The units are shown in Table 10-1.

The central objectives of our project can be defined as follows: (a) How widely were we able to carry out the different activities involved in our therapeutic orientation and what kind of patients did we treat? (b) What effects did the therapeutic orientation on the whole and the different therapeutic activities involved in it have on the prognoses of the patients? (c) What experiences did we have concerning indications for the different therapeutic activities? (d)What was the global "model" of therapeutic activities we ultimately constructed, and what kind of resources are required for an optimal implementation of the different activities?

This presentation will mainly deal with the first and the second of these objectives.

**Table 10-1.   Community Psychiatric Treatment Units of
the Mental Health District of the City of Turku**

(a)	Hospitals*		
	Clinic of Psychiatry (University Hospital)	111	beds
	Clinic of Psychiatry (University Hospital)	18	day patients
	Kupittaa Hospital	364	beds
	Other hospitals outside the Turku area		
	(only chronic patients)	139	beds

*3.7 beds per 1,000 inhabitants

(b)	Open Care Turku Mental Health Office	1.2 staff members per 10,000 inhabitants
	Clinic of Psychiatry aftercare activity	accomplished by staff members working at the wards
	Psychiatric Outpatient Clinic of the University Central Hospital (General Hospital	6 staff members primarily active in liaison psychiatry

Patient Series and Its Diagnostic Classification

In accordance with the action research nature of the project, we defined the diagnostic criteria for inclusion in the series
relatively widely. The most central criterion was the presence of
definite psychotic symptoms of the schizophrenic type indica-
tive of a disintegration of the previous functional level of the
personality. We consider this accordant with the genuine Bleulerian tradition, which maintains that the primary psychic disorder in schizophrenia consists of an elementary weakness in
functional integrity, which pertains to both drives and emotions
on the one hand and associations on the other.[2, 3]

**Table 10-2. Diagnostic Distribution
of the Patient Sample**

Diagnostic Group	Age Range			
	16–25	26–35	36–45	Total
Typical Schizophrenia	24	22	10	56
Schizophreniform Psychosis	1	5	4	10
Schizo-Affective Psychosis	3	8	3	14
Borderline Psychosis	6	10	4	20
Total	34	45	21	100

At the same time, we divided the series into four diagnostic subcategories (see Table 10-2), the largest of which was the group of typical schizophrenias with more persistent symptoms of the kind suggested by Langfeldt,[4] which comprised 56 patients. As far as we can see, the diagnostic limits of the group approximate to the criteria of "schizophrenic disorder" proposed in the American DSM III classification,[5] though they remain slightly wider. The main difference lies in the fact that our diagnostic system did not include the kind of strict criterion based on a long duration of the disorder that was included in the DSM III classification. Our other diagnostic subcategories were schizophreniform psychosis, schizo-affective psychosis, and borderline psychosis.[6, 7] When discussing the prognostic findings, we consider separately the entire series on the one hand and the group of typical schizophrenias on the other.

During the course of the work, we also made another diagnostic classification, which had psychodynamic premises and was based on an assessment of the disturbance of the patient's ego functions, i.e. the degree and duration of disintegration and its dynamic meaningfulness. We will here also briefly describe this ego-psychologic classification of ours, because it turned out to be significant in the subsequent analyses. Table 10-3 shows the classification in relation to our diagnostic subcategories.

The group of imminent ego disintegration consisted of the patients whose psychotic condition was characterized by ominous, imminent fragmentation of the ego function, but who were not in a massive psychotic condition. This group largely

Table 10-3.   Distribution of the Patients According to
the Ego-Psychologic Group

| Ego-Psychologic Group | Diagnostic Group | | | | |
	Typ. Sch	S-Form Psych	S-Aff. Psych	Bord. Psych	In Total
Imminent Disintegration	0*	2	1	18*	21
Acute Disintegration	9**	6***	11*	2***	28
Regressive Disintegration	29*	0***	2	0*	31
Paranoid Disintegration	18*	2	0***	0***	20
Total	56	10	14	20	100

* = p < .001,   ** = p < .01,   *** = p < .05

corresponds to borderline psychoses. The symptoms were of
clearly defensive significance in protecting the patient against
internal anxiety and more profound disintegration of the personality.

The group of acute ego disintegration consisted of the patients whose psychotic condition developed relatively suddenly
and was massive. The symptoms were rather characterized by
decompensation of the previous psychic balance than by defensive significance.

The group of regressive ego disintegration consisted of the
patients whose illness was clearly related to persistent and serious difficulties of adjustment in interpersonal relationships and
social coping. The psychotic symptoms generally appeared
gradually and slowly, though they could be sudden in some
cases, but even the patients with a sudden onset of symptoms
had had conspicuous difficulties in their prepsychotic adjustment. The psychotic symptoms were profound, and although
they were of internal defensive significance for the patients at
the psychotic level, they generally interfered badly with social
coping.

The group of paranoid ego disintegration, finally, consisted of the patients whose psychotic development was domi-
nated by rigid, typically paranoid formations, which, from the
psychodynamic point of view, signify a projective way of solving psychological problems. The disintegration of the ego was

Table 10-4. Accomplished Psychotherapeutic Activities According to Five-Year Follow-Up

Mode of Treatment	Number of Patients	
Crisis Treatment in the Beginning Phase	28	28
Intensive Individual Therapy	26	57
Minor Individual Therapy	31	
Intensive Family Therapy	15	25
Minor Family Therapy	10	
Supportive Contact with Family Member(s)	40	
Intensive Group Therapy	1	2
Minor Group Therapy	1	
Intensive Treatment in a Psychother. Community	25	
Crisis Treatment in a Psychother. Community	21	56
Minor Treatment in a Psychother. Community	18	
No Psychotherapeutic Treatment Mode		20

less generalized than in the previous group, and the patients were better able to cope socially.

Both of these classifications, the one based on the classical diagnostic critetia and the one based on ego-psychological premises, turned out to be significant in our subsequent analyses. They supplemented each other in, e.g., the analyses of the implementation of different modes of therapy.

Course of Study and Methods

Our original team consisted of four members, of whom three (Alanen, Räkköläinen, and Rasimus) were working in the Clinic of Psychiatry, while one (Laakso) belonged to the staff of the Turku Mental Health Office.[8, 9] A psychiatric basic examination was carried out on all the patients; it included separate interviews of the patient, on the one hand, and the members of his family, on the other, as well as the deliberation of a therapeutic plan. Since the implementation of the therapies remained at the responsibility of the different units, not all of them were carried out in accordance with our plans, but were influenced by several selective factors emanating from among both the therapeutic staff and the patients. The question of what kind of patients are given psychotherapeutic treatments and what kind of patients are not is also a highly relevant object of study.

The first follow-up examination of individuals and families similar to the basic examination was carried out by our team after 2 years, and another similar follow-up examination was undertaken 5 years after the admission for therapy. The findings to be presented here are based on the psychiatric basic examination as well as the psychiatric 5 year follow-up.

The data acquired in the basic examination were recorded on a 163-item form. On the basis of that form, we constructed more than 40 clinical and psychosocial background variables.*

In the 5-year follow-up examination we analyzed the correlations between these background variables and the implementation of the different therapies, as well as the connections between the background variables and the treatment variables constructed from the implementation of the therapies, on one hand, and the prognoses of our patients, on the other.

The statistical analyses were based on crosstabulations of the different groups of variables, on one hand, and logistic regression analysis, on the other. The latter method was applied to study the implementation of the different modes of therapy as well as the variables explaining the prognosis.

The lack of a control series naturally limited the conclusions that can be made on the basis of our findings concerning the outcome of the psychotherapeutic orientation. The most central starting point here was the comparison between the prognosis of the "group of psychotherapy cases" emerging from our series (cf. later, it included 54 of the patients covered in the 5-year follow-up) and the prognosis of the patients not included in this group and mainly treated with pharmacotherapy (41 patients in the 5-year follow-up).

---

*Information about the background variables, the treatment variables, and the prognostic variables used in the analyses may be obtained from the authors.

Implementation of therapies

The organization of the Turku Mental Health District was quite heavily hospital-oriented in the late 1970s: only 21 of our 100 patients were admitted for treatment via an outpatient unit, and for no more than 17 of these 21 was the outpatient unit the first therapeutic unit. The inpatient wards of the Clinic of Psychiatry were the first therapeutic unit for 54 patients and the day hospital ward for 5, while 24 patients were first treated in the Kupittaa Hospital, the other psychiatric hospital of the district.

Nevertheless, we endeavored to develop the therapeutic orientation particularly toward outpatient therapy. When we classified the psychotherapeutic treatments carried out during the 5-year follow-up period, we only included in the classes of individual, family, and group therapy the treatments that had been given, at least partially, within the outpatient system. The therapeutic relationships restricted to an inpatient ward were considered as included in treatments given in a psychotherapeutic community. This procedure is related to our notion that the crucial part of the psychotherapy of a schizophrenic patient should always take place with the patient living in his normal environment, where he is supported and encouraged to analyze his problems with the therapist. Table 10-4 shows a summary of the psychotherapeutic activities carried out during the 5 follow-up years. The criteria it shows for the different modes of therapy were set on the basis of the duration of the treatment and the number of therapeutic sessions. The following criteria were used:

Initial intervention in crisis: Help given in a situation of psychotic crisis by means of rapidly initiated and frequent therapeutic visits with individual or family and environmental orientation on an outpatient basis or through brief hospitalization.

Intensive individual therapy: At least 2 years of therapy, at least 80 therapeutic sessions.

Less intensive individual therapy: At least 6 months of therapy, at least 12 sessions.

Intensive family therapy: At least 6 months of therapy, at least 12 joint sessions.

Less intensive family therapy: At least 3 joint sessions.

Supportive contact to family member(s): Contact with the patient's family or a member of his family beyond the actual study period for the purpose of supporting the family during the patient's treatment.

Intensive group therapy: At least 1 year of therapy, at least 24 sessions.

Less intensive group therapy: At least 6 sessions.

Intensive therapy in psychotherapeutic community: At least 3 months of therapy; a) a personal patient-therapist contact; b) situational exploration of the family and the living milieu; and c) involvement of the patient in the group and community processes of the ward.

Intervention in crisis in psychotherapeutic community: Shorter but active community therapy in a critical situation, including exploration of and intervention in the patient's family and/or social environment.

Less intensive community therapy: Treatment in a therapeutic community that was not in all respects equally active and extensive as described above, but involved an empathic approach to the patient and his participation in the ward's group and community functions.

As regards outpatient therapy, the units of the mental health district were responsible for 73 percent of the individual, family, and group therapies carried out. Of the therapies, 22 percent were accomplished in the private sector, which was, quite intentionally, utilized as supplementary to the inadequate resources of the public sector.

The occupational categories of the therapists in charge of the individual, family, and group therapies, and the number of cases they were responsible for, are shown in Table 10-5. The number is higher than the total number of therapies, because some therapies were carried out successively by two or several therapists.

What attracts attention in the table is the fact that the ther-

Table 10-5.   Therapist's Occupational Groups.*

Professional Category	Number of Therapists	Number of Cases
Psychiatrists	13	24
Resident Physicians in Training	10	22
Psychologists	8	12
Nurses Specialized in Psych. Nursing	13	41
Nurses	1	1
Psychiatric Aides	3	3
Social Workers	4	7
Total	52	110

*Only eight therapists had formal psychotherapeutic training; 39 therapists had on-the-job training and long-term therapy supervision

Table 10-6.   Implementation of Intensive Individual Therapy: Variables Influencing the Selective Processes (Logistic Regression Analysis).

Explaining Variables	R*	p
All Patients		
Insight Ability (yes/no)	3.42	0.000
Acting Out Behavior (no/yes)	4.86	0.000
Beginning of Symptoms (acute/slow)	2.83	0.008
Neurotic Symptoms (yes/no)	2.06	0.015
Unemployed (no/yes)	3.38	0.038
Typical Schizophrenics		
Duration of Symptoms Before Treatment Admission (>1 mo/<1 mo)	3.00	0.009
Mother's Severe Personality Disorder (no/yes)	2.59	0.061

*R = risk; i.e. the relative probability of those differentiated by the explaining variable to be included in the response group

apies were carried out by as many as 52 therapists. The therapists were most often specialized psychiatrists and specialized nurses, both of which numbered 13.

Intensive individual therapy was clearly the mode of psychotherapy longest in duration in our series. The mean number of therapeutic sessions for the 26 patients receiving this mode of treatment was 163. Despite the name we use, the intensity of the therapy was variable: although there were often as many as two or three sessions weekly at the initial stages, the average frequency of sessions generally came down to one per week during the course of the therapy. Table 10-6 indicates that intensive individual therapy was selectively given to patients—or could best be given to patients—whose primary insight ability was better than average. The explaining variable second in importance was the absence of acting-out behavior: according to our experience, the individuals showing acting-out behavior were the ones who most frequently discontinued individual therapy. The group was further characterized by some other clinical or psychosocially favorable background variables.

In the group of typical schizophrenias, intensive individual therapy was given to 14 patients, or 25 percent, which is more or less exactly the same percentage as in the entire series. A separate analysis of this group of patients showed an absence of serious personality disorders in the mother to emerge as one explaining variable.

The family orientation in our therapeutic approach was carried out most extensively and probably most successfully through supportive contacts to the family members. The fact that the therapist met the family and created a favorable relationship with its members was clearly highly useful for the implementation of individual therapies, and the families often also contacted the therapist or another member of the treatment team later, the patient being aware of it.

Joint family therapy sessions were attended by 25 patients altogether, if we take into account both the intensive and the less intensive therapies. Of these, 11 were conjoint therapies of the primary family, and 15, couple therapies of the patients and his or her spouse (one patient was given both forms of therapy). Table 10-7 can be interpreted in such a way that a particularly large number of very ill, regressively disintegrated patients were

**Table 10-7.   Implementation of Family Therapy:
Variables Influencing the Selective Processes
(Logistic Regression Analysis).**

Explaining Variables	R	p
All Patients		
Ego-Psychologic Group of Regressive Disintegration (yes/no)	2.05	0.042
Psychosexual Development ("normal"/"abnormal")	1.94	0.012
Earlier Psychiatric Treatment (yes/no)	1.90	0.067
Typical Schizophrenics		
Depressive Symptoms (yes/no)	3.75	0.006
Psychosexual Development ("normal"/"abnormal")	2.52	0.050

**Table 10-8.   Implementation of Treatment in
Psychotherapeutic Community: Variables Influencing
the Selective Process (Logistic Regression Analysis):**

Explaining Variables	R	p
All Patients		
Group of Regressive Disintegration (yes/no)	2.58	0.001
Sex (female/male)	2.09	0.001
Group of Imminent Disintegration (no/yes)	3.36	0.031
Refusing Treatment in the Beginning Phase (no/yes)	1.90	0.049
Typical Schizophrenics		
Group of Regressive Disintegration (yes/no)	2.66	0.002
Quality of Interpersonal Relationships Outside of the Primary Family (not stable/stable)	1.77	0.013
Depressive Symptoms (yes/no)	1.78	0.030

selected for the conjoint therapy of the primary family—the group including a greater than average number of patients previously treated in a child-psychiatric unit or by private psychiatrists—while the married patients given couple therapy were the ones with "normal" psychosexual development compared with the whole series. Intensive therapy or intervention in crisis in a psychotherapeutic community (Table 10-8) was also given to several patients belonging to the group of regressive ego disintegration.

Table 10-9 indicates that the selection of the patients into the psychotherapy group was most notably influenced by the first therapeutic unit. The patients first treated in the Clinic of Psychiatry and the Turku Mental Health Office became psychotherapy cases with almost threefold probability, compared with the patients of the Kupittaa Hospital.

The explaining variable second in importance in the whole series is the accumulation of patients with regressive ego disintegration in the group of psychotherapy cases. Among the typical schizophrenic patients this parameter did not emerge as an explaining variable, though it had a remarkable statistical correlation with the psychotherapy cases (p=.014). We can hence claim that these patients are well within the reach of therapy, unlike the patients with paranoid ego disintegration, who had a significant negative correlation with the group of psychotherapy cases in the whole series (p=.034) and a marginal negative correlation even in the group of typical schizophrenics (p=.058). Of the classical diagnostic subcategories, the only one to display a statistical correlation with the psychotherapy cases was the group of schizophreniform psychoses, which was largely excluded from the group of psychotherapy cases (p=.016). Of the typical schizophrenic patients, 57 percent belonged to the group of psychotherapy cases, which percentage is equal to that seen in the total series.

These correlations between the group of psychotherapy cases and the diagnostic background variables indicate that the group included relatively more seriously ill patients than the rest of the series. The number of patients with regressive ego disintegration was about twofold in the group of psychotherapy cases, compared with the remaining part of the series, while only one-fifth of the patients with schizophreniform psychoses with a good prognosis belonged to the group of psychotherapy cases. This clinical difference, however, is partly leveled off by the notable presence of some other, favorable background variables in the selection into the psychotherapy group. As is shown by Table 10-9, these variables included the patient's tendency to symbiotic reliance and the patient's being employed upon

**Table 10-9.   Belonging to the Group of Psychotherapy
Cases: Variables Influencing the Selective Processes
(Logistic Regression Analysis):**

Explaining Variables	R	p
All Patients		
First Therapeutic Unit (Clinic of psychiatry or open care/Kupittaa Hospital)	2.63	0.000
Group of Regressive Disintegration (yes/no)	1.97	0.009
Symbiotic Contact Mode (yes/no)	1.69	0.015
Unemployed (yes/no)	1.97	0.014
Typical Schizophrenics		
First Therapeutic Unit (Clinic of psychiatry or open care/Kupittaa Hospital)	2.72	0.024
Beginning of Symptoms (acute/slow)	1.98	0.021
Refusing Treatment in the Beginning Phase (no/yes)	1.78	0.015

**Table 10-10.   Lack of any Mode of Psychotherapeutic
Treatment: Influence of Background Variables
(Logistic Regression Analysis).**

Explaining Variables	R	p
All Patients		
Depressive Symptoms (no/yes)	3.27	0.005
Basic Education (elementary school/more)	6.00	0.005
Sex (male/female)	3.875	0.050
Typical Schizophrenics		
Ego-Psychologic Group of Paranoid Disintegration (yes/no)	4.92	0.004
Depressive Symptoms (no/yes)	5.29	0.001
Alcohol or Other Addiction (yes/no)	2.93	0.108
Unemployed (yes/no)	3.32	0.124

admission in the total series, and a relatively acute onset of the psychosis and a lack of negativism towards therapy in the group of typical schizophrenic patients.

What about patients completely excluded from the psychotherapeutic treatments? We also made a logistic regression analysis on the group of patients who were not given even any of the less intensive psychotherapeutic treatments shown in Table 10-3 (with the exception of support given to the family, which could take place even when the patient had not been met personally). Table 10-10 indicates that the patients most difficult to reach by means of therapy were particularly those without depressive symptoms who used paranoid defenses as well as individuals whose social conditions were poorer than the average (low level of basic education, unemployment, alcohol problems). The probability of men belonging to this group of patients was nearly fourfold that of women. It might be pointed out that although some of these factors were discussed in explaining the selection of the first therapeutic unit, the first therapeutic unit did not emerge as an explaining variable in this analysis.

Of our 100 patients, 98 received neuroleptic medication at some stage of their treatment, though many only for a short period. During the last 3 follow-up years, 40 percent of our patients were completely without pharmacotherapy.

We divided the patients into two groups on the basis of the amount of medication they consumed during the whole follow-up period. The explaining variables of the group given more medication are shown in Table 11-11. It is interesting that this analysis, in addition to emphasizing the group of regressively disintegrated patients and the first therapeutic unit, also brings up the assessment of whether the patient has inadequately understanding or hostile relatives in his family environment as made in the basic examination. In the group of typical schizophrenic patients, this assessment is the most important variable explaining abundant pharmacotherapy. The finding is parallel to the conclusions made by Leff and Vaughn[10] in Britain, using a different research strategy.

Our team considered it significant that the group of psychotherapy cases had a clearly significant positive correlation with the presence of medication during the first 2 follow-up

**Table 10-11.   Larger Neuroleptic Medication during the
Follow-Up Years: Influence of Background Variables
(Logistic Regression Analysis)**

Explaining Variables	R	p
All Patients		
Group of Regressive Disintegration (yes/no)	2.26	0.000
First Therapeutic Unit		
(Kupittaa Hospital/open care)	1.66	0.003
(Kupittaa Hospital/Clinic of Psychiatry)	2.05	
Hostile or Insufficiently Understanding Relatives		
(yes/no)	1.58	0.001
Typical Schizophrenics		
Hostile or Insufficiently Understanding Relatives		
(yes/no)	1.88	0.001
Group of Regressive Disintegration (yes/no)	1.57	0.003
Sex (male/female)	1.53	0.008

years, while during the last 3 years of follow-up the correlation with the amount of medication was negative, though only at a marginally significant level. Only one patient in our psychotherapy group continued to have high-dose neuroleptic medication corresponding to at least 300 mg of chlorpromazine daily during the last 3 years of follow-up, while 10 other patients in our series had such high-dose medication.

PROGNOSIS AND CONTRIBUTING FACTORS

We were able to acquire data on the condition of 95 patients in our 5-year follow-up study. Of the remaining patients, three had died, all of them by suicide.

Only 30 percent of our patients were found to have psychotic symptoms at the follow-up (Table 10-12). The corresponding figure for the group of typical schizophrenic patients was 50 percent. Transient manifestation of psychotic symptoms, however, was considered possible in some nonpsychotic patients.

**Table 10-12.   Presence of Psychotic Symptoms at the
Time of the Five-Year Follow-Up
(Percent of the Number of Patients)**

| Diagnostic Group | Presence of Symptoms | | | |
| | Present | | Absent | |
	Marked	Mild	Potential	Definite
Typical Schizophrenia (n = 51)	18	33	16	33
		51		49
Schizophreniform Psych. (n = 9)	0	0	11	89
Schizo-Affect. Psychosis (n = 12)	0	0	17	83
Borderline Psychosis (n = 20)	0	10	10	80
Total (n = 92)	9	20	15	55
		30		70

On the whole, the clinical prognosis of our patients can be considered relatively good in the light of the figures here presented, which also is shown by comparison with most studies with corresponding series and follow-up periods.[11-14]

The prognosis of working capacity for our patients must be considered somewhat more pessimistic than their clinical prognosis. At the end of the follow-up period, only 43 percent of the patients were fully capable of working normally (Table 10-13). The corresponding figure for the group of typical schizophrenics being 33 percent. The difference between this group and the other diagnostic groups was smaller than that found in the clinical prognosis.

It is particularly appropriate to discuss here the effects of the therapies carried out as well as of the clinical and psychosocial background variables on the prognosis of the patients. We analyzed the prognosis multidimensionally. Here we can examine four prognostic variables, which simultaneously reveal the changes or the developmental tendency visible in the condition of the patients during the 5 years between the basic examination and the latter follow-up examination. They are: disappearance of psychotic symptoms, decrease of the nuclear symptoms of schizophrenia, increase of insight, and working capacity. Of

**Table 10-13. Working Capacity of the Patients at the
Time of the Five-Year Follow-Up
(Percent of the Number of Patients)**

Diagnostic Groups	Working Capacity		
	None	Diminished	Full
Typical Schizophrenia (n = 54)	47	20	33
Schizophreniform Psych. (n = 9)	0	22	78
Schizo-Affective Psychosis (n = 12)	25	25	50
Borderline Psychosis (n = 20)	10	40	50
Total (n = 95)	32	25	43

these prognostic variables, two are clinical, the third is psycho-dynamic, and the fourth psychosocial.

We again applied the logistic regression analysis, examining simultaneously the effects of the background variables and the therapeutic variables on the changes noted in the prognosis. The following treatment variables were used: inclusion in the group of psychotherapy cases, intensive individual therapy, family therapy (both intensive and less intensive), intensive treatment or intervention in crisis in a psychotherapeutic community, and the amount of neuroleptic drug therapy (higher or lower than the average).

Since all of the patients had psychotic symptoms upon admission, the disappearance of psychotic symptoms was measured by noting which of the patients had manifest psychotic symptoms at the end of the 5-year follow-up period and which did not (the distributions are shown in Table 10-12).

Logistic regression analysis (Table 10-14) discriminated as explaining variables two clinical background variables whose significance is clearly understandable: exclusion of the patient from the diagnostic category of typical schizophrenics, and acute onset of his symptoms. Less than average neuroleptic medication emerged as the third explaining variable. The significance of this variable, too, appears understandable at least at first sight: after all, abundant medication was indicated for the more seriously ill patients. It could have been expected, however, that the significance of this factor would have decreased in a separate

**Table 10-14.   Disappearance of Psychotic Symptoms at
the Time of the Five-Year Follow-Up: Influence of
Background and/or Treatment Variables
(Logistic Regression).**

Explaining Variables	R	p
All Patients		
Diagnostic Group		
Typical Schizophrenia (no/yes)	1.94	0.000
Beginning of Symptoms (acute/slow)	1.58	0.001
Drug Treatment (little/much)	1.78	0.020
Typical Schizophrenics		
Drug Treatment (little/much)	2.17	0.008
Beginning of Symptoms (acute/slow)	2.63	0.035

analysis of the group of typical schizophrenic patients, for whom
continuous pharmacologically sufficient medication is generally
considered an appropriate form of treatment. But this was not
what happened: a separate analysis of the nuclear group of patients revealed less than average medication as the variable most
closely related to the disappearance of psychotic symptoms.

None of the other treatment variables emerged as explaining variables in this analysis. When examined separately, however, intensive individual therapy had a significant ($p<.05$)
positive correlation with the disappearance of psychotic symptoms both in the total series and in the group of typical schizophrenic patients. Inclusion in the group of psychotherapy cases
had a statistically similar ($p= .029$) correlation with the disappearance of symptoms in the group of typical schizophrenics,
but not in the whole series.

Our analysis of the decrease of the nuclear symptoms of
schizophrenia supplemented the analysis of the disappearance
of psychotic symptoms in that it demonstrated even the favorable development that had taken place in the more seriously ill
patients. Improvement on a three-step scale (0–1, 2–3, 4 or more
nuclear symptoms) had taken place in the case of 58 patients,
while 16 patients displayed no such improvement. The patients

Table 10-15. Decrease of the Nuclear Symptoms of Schizophrenia during the Five-Year Follow-Up Period; Influence of Background and/or Treatment Variables (Logistic Regression)

Explaining Variables	R	p
All Patients		
Diagnostic Group Typical Schizophrenia (no/yes)	1.41	0.002
Separated from the Primary Family (yes/no)	1.39	0.006
Intensive Individual Therapy (yes/no)	1.33	0.004
Typical Schizophrenics		
Separated from the Primary Family (yes/no)	1.61	0.011
Psychotherapy Case (yes/no)	1.63	0.004

who had only been diagnosed for one nuclear symptom at the time of the basic examination were left out of this comparison.

The most marked explaining variable in the whole series even now is the exclusion of the patient from the group of typical schizophrenics (Table 10-15). The explaining variable second in importance is separation from the primary family already noted at the time of the basic examination, which also retains its position when the analysis is restricted to the patients with typical schizophrenia. It is hence a significant predictive factor for alleviation of the severity of psychosis. In addition to these, one treatment variable emerges as an explaining variable in both cases, namely intensive individual therapy in the whole series and inclusion in the group of psychotherapy cases in the group of typical schizophrenic. The analysis thus clearly demonstrates the favorable effect of psychotherapy on the clinical prognosis of the patients in the schizophrenia group. Neuroleptic medication was not equally significant in this analysis as in the analysis concerning the complete disappearance of psychotic symptoms. The increase of insight was also analyzed with a three-step scale. The scale was relatively simple, and therefore straightforward and easy to use: the patient either lacked any insight into his own role in the development of his problems and/or symptoms, or he had some insight into it, or he saw his problems and symptoms as part of himself and endeavored to solve them. The insight was considered to have increased if the patient had improved on the scale during the period between the basic examination and the follow-up examination. Altogether 27 patients exhibited such an improvement (including 13 typical schizophrenics), while no improvement had taken place in the case of 65 (41 typical schizophrenics). The 3 patients estimated to have the best possible insight grade even at the basic examination stage were left out of this analysis.

The effect of psychotherapy on the increase of insight turned out to be of crucial importance (Table 10-16). In the total series, inclusion in the group of psychotherapy cases as well as intensive treatment or intervention in crisis in a psychotherapeutic community had a clearly significant correlation with the increase of insight ($p<.01$), while intensive individual therapy had an almost significant ($p<.02$) correlation. In the group of typical schizophrenics, the correlations of inclusion in the group of psychotherapy cases and intensive individual therapy increased even further, being highly significant ($p<.001$), while the correlation for psychotherapeutic treatment community remained at its previous level. Family therapy did not correlate with the increase of insight, while abundant medication seemed to have a negative effect, particularly in the group of typical schizophrenics ($p<.05$). Logistic regression analysis showed that most notable variable explaining the improvement of insight to be inclusion in the group of psychotherapy cases in the whole series, and intensive individual therapy in the group of typical schizophrenics. The variable second in importance in both analyses was the lack of alcohol or addiction problems.

It was obvious that the psychosocial conditions, particularly the unemployment situation, affected the working capacity of our patients. This is clearly shown in Table 10-17, where the factors explaining the working capacity are given for the whole series and the group of typical schizophrenias. The effect of unemployment clearly dominates in the former analysis, and all the other explaining variables are also psychosocial background variables. In the group of typical schizophrenias, a lower than average neuroleptic treatment during the follow-up period correlates clearly with the maintenance of working capacity.

Table 10-16. Increase of Insight During the Five-Year Follow-Up Period: Influence of Background and/or Treatment Variables (Logistic Regression)

Explaining Variables	R	p
All Patients		
Psychotherapy Case (yes/no)	3.53	0.001
Alcohol or Other Addiction (no/yes)	3.22	0.008
Socially Deviating Family Background (yes/no)	1.86	0.008
Typical Schizophrenics		
Intensive Individual Therapy (yes/no)	4.57	0.001
Alcohol or Other Addiction (yes/no)	6.47	0.004

Table 10-17. Working Capacity at the Time of the Five-Year Follow-Up: Influence of Background and/or Treatment Variables (Logistic Regression).

Explaining Variables	R	p
All Patients		
Unemployed (no/yes)	10.66	0.000
Occupational Identity (formed/not formed)	1.81	0.003
Basic Education (more/elementary)	1.56	0.008
Sex (female/male)	1.66	0.023
Hostile or Insufficiently Understanding Relatives (no/yes)	2.03	0.031
Typical Schizophrenics		
Neuroleptic Treatment (little/much)	4.78	0.000
Sex (female/male)	4.38	0.013
Basic Education (more/elementary)	2.11	0.006
Alcohol or Other Addiction (no/yes)	9.17	0.079

The effect of psychosocial factors such as the state of unemployment in all probability accounted for the discrepancy found between the clinical and psychosocial outcome of our patients. They also contribute to the finding according to which the difference between the outcome of working capacity of the patients included in the nuclear group and those of other diagnostic groups is here smaller than the difference concerning the improvement of psychotic symptoms. The psychosocial outcome of female patients was clearly better than that of male patients, especially those with a lower than average basic education, and lacking occupational identity. The negative effect of relatives' hostile or nonunderstanding attitudes toward the patient also turned out to be one of the explaining variables in the analysis of the whole patients series.

But what about the psychotherapy variables? Even if the inclusion in the group of psychotherapy cases did not emerge in the logistic regression as an explaining variable, it correlated significantly (P<.05) with the maintenance of working capacity in the total series. When the analysis was restricted to the group of typical schizophrenia, the correlation turned out to be clearly significant (p= .002; of the 32 typical schizophrenics belonging to the group of psychotherapy cases, 16 had a normal working capacity, while only 2 of the other 22 typical schizophrenics were able to work normally). Intensive individual therapy as well as intensive treatment or intervention in crisis in a psychotherapeutic community had a significant correlation with the maintenance of working capacity in the group of typical schizophrenias.

DISCUSSION

Our most essential conclusion is that the follow-up study gives a favorable overall view of the meaningfulness of developing a global psychotherapeutic approach to treating schizophrenia. In the light of our prognostic analyses, the development of the patients included in the group of psychotherapy cases was clearly more favorable than the development of the patients not given psychotherapy. Apart from the variable consisting of the group of psychotherapy cases, two therapeutic variables pertaining to certain modes of psychotherapy, i.e. intensive individual therapy and intensive treatment in a psychotherapeutic community, or intervention in crisis in a psychotherapeutic community, had statistical correlations with a favorable prognosis, most distinctly with the increase of insight and clearly also with clinical and psychosocial prognostic variables.

The significance particularly of the correlations between the group of psychotherapy cases representing the global therapeutic approach and the prognostic variables increases when the development of the typical schizophrenic patients is examined separately from the whole series. It therefore seems that the typical schizophrenic patients benefited from the psychotherapeutic treatment at least as much as the patients not included in this nuclear group.

As was suggested at the beginning, we are aware of the restrictions of our developmental project as a prognostic investigation in comparison with the result of "controlled" studies of therapeutic outcome. There are two distinctive factors susceptible to criticism: there is no control material and the team members themselves make the assessments in the follow-up examination.

The first of these shortcomings is partly compensated by our opportunity of making comparisons between patients given psychotherapy and those who did not receive psychotherapeutic treatment. As was previously pointed out, the group of psychotherapy cases included a relatively greater proportion of seriously ill patients, diagnostically speaking, than the rest of the series. On the other hand, the group of psychotherapy cases was notably characterized by some other background factors that contributed favorably to a good outcome of therapy.

The risk of subjectivity in the assessments was approached by instituting a follow-up examination carried out by an independent psychiatrist parallel to the examination made by the team at the time of the 2-year follow-up. This examiner had not previously met any of our patients, but was familiar with the nature of our therapeutic approach. It turned out that her prognostic assessments were clearly more favorable on an average than the assessments made by the team, particularly notably so in the clinical evaluations. It seems that this was most crucially due to the fact that the team members had been familiar with the patients for a longer period and had information on them from sources other than the single patient interview, on which the independent examiner had to base her assessments. The mutual correlation between the assessments was of the order of 0.6–0.7 for the clinical prognosis variables and 0.5 or more for the other prognostic subareas compared.It can further be pointed out that the assessments made by the independent examiner also resulted, almost regularly, in more significant findings concerning the favorable prognosis of the patients given psychotherapy as compared with the other patients than did the evaluations by our team members.[7]

The independent examination was not repeated at the time of the 5-year follow-up, because we deemed it in no way essential for providing additional information to meet our goals.

To what extent did our expectations and objectives pertaining to our developmental work come true?

We are satisfied with the number of therapeutic activities carried out, although the optimal realization of the needs of the patients and their families was not yet reached. The quantitative staff resources of our clinic and the entire Turku Mental Health District are relatively modest.

But even the extent of therapeutic activities now achieved seems to indicate that qualitative resources are clearly more crucial than quantitative resources for the development of the psychotherapeutic treatments of schizophrenic patients. In this respect, the Turku Mental Health District with its university teaching hospital is in a better than average position, which does not, however, mean that a corresponding development could not take place under ordinary circumstances. As a matter of fact, we currently try to develop this kind of therapeutic orientation in several other mental health districts in Finland within a national program for developing the treatment of schizophrenia.

Our experiences of the different modes of therapy were most favorable for the psychotherapeutic communities on the one hand and for intensive individual therapy on the other.

Despite the criticism of the psychiatric hospital institution and the risks of excessive hospital orientation—which were mentioned previously—the ward communities with an open and empathic atmosphere are of pivotal significance for the psychotherapeutic treatment of schizophrenic patients. One important requirement for the overall meaningfulness of the therapeutic activities is that units do not consider themselves self-sufficient, but extend their activities outside their own limits, endeavoring to make contacts with the patients' living milieu outside the hospital and to support the patients upon return to their own living environment. The planning of further treatment is also included among their tasks.

The patients selected for intensive individual therapies were mostly those who, even initially, had some insight into their problems. The therapies of these patients were successfully conducted even by therapists who had not been given actual psychotherapeutic training, but received regular supervision, e.g. by specialized nurses with both empathic skills and practical experience in the problems typical of schizophrenic patients.

These favorable experiences give rise to some more general conclusions. First of all, we want to suggest that—despite opposite notions—the outcome of long-term individual therapy in the group of schizophrenic patients is often good when the therapy is given selectively to suitable patients. Regardless of the clinical severity or the diagnosis of the illness, the suitable patients are those who tend to establish a reliant contact with the therapist, who are even initially motivated to analyze their problems, and who have no tendency to acting-out behavior. It would be important that at least the patients of this kind could be guaranteed a possibility to have the therapy they need notably more often than is the case at the present.

Secondly, we should not underestimate the importance of individual therapies based on relatively infrequent sessions, but an empathic and confidential therapeutic relationship, for the treatment of psychotic patients. The significance of the therapeutic relationship as such, as well as the personal properties of the therapist, are especially important in this group of patients, compared with the more technically oriented psychoanalytic therapies of neurotic patients. Therapeutic "holding,"[15, 16] which satisfies empathically the patient's symbiotic needs, but also supports his growth into differentiation, forms the basis for such therapeutic relationships. Serious transference crises, which frequently result in a discontinuation of the therapy, are easier to avoid in this kind of therapy than in more intensive, psychoanalytically oriented therapies.

In the light of our findings, the results of family therapy remained much below the corresponding results of individual therapy, which is largely the reverse of the views presented in some other papers.[17] It is therefore necessary to underscore that our findings do not do justice to family therapy in comparison with individual and community therapy for several reasons. Family therapy was given to fewer patients, and we had to include both the intensive and the less intensive therapies in our family therapy variable, unlike in the case of individual therapy and community therapy.

The other reason for our findings on family therapy included the lesser changes of training and supervision available for family therapy than for individual therapy at the time our patients were admitted. Moreover, the family therapies of primary families were carried out among very seriously ill patients. The results of couple therapy were better, but do not stand out in our statistical analysis.

In the present study the significance of the psychodynamics of the family system was also shown by the emergence of some background factors associated with it—and defined at the basic examination stage—as variables explaining the prognosis in several different analyses. This can also be interpreted as an indication for increasing family-centered activities in the further development of the treatment of schizophrenic patients.

The correlations between psychopharmacologic treatment and the prognosis appeared as negative in our statistical analyses. This does not do justice to the significance of pharmacologic treatment in the overall therapeutic situation: as was pointed out, nearly all of our patients were given neuroleptic treatment at least initially in the therapy. During the first 2 follow-up years, the psychopharmacologic treatment and the psychotherapies correlated positively, but during the last 3 years of follow-up a negative correlation emerged. Medication was used as a supplementary means in the psychotherapeutic approach. It was useful especially at the early stages of the therapy, but was often discontinued as soon as the patient was considered to manage without it.

Should the negative correlation between the amount of medication and the poor prognosis be interpreted in such a way that the most seriously ill patients need more medication and also have a poorer prognosis? Undoubtedly, this is partly true. But another reason appears to be that the patients with heavy medication did not receive psychotherapeutic treatment as often as the other patients; in other words, the favorable effect of psychotherapy was lacking in their case. The cases of some individual patients also gave rise to an assumption that the directly passivizing effect of medication contributed to their poor prognosis. Of the prognostic variables, massive medication had the strongest negative correlation with the maintenance of working ability, which may lend support to this assumption.

REFERENCES

1. Alanen, Y. O. The psychotherapeutic care of schizophrenic patients in a community psychiatric setting. In M. H. Lader (Ed.) Studies in schizophrenia, *British Journal of Psychiatry,* 1975, Special Publication No. *10,* 86–93.

2. Bleuler, E. *Dementia praecox order die Gruppe der Schizophrenien.* Leipzig-Wien: Deuricke, 1911.

3. Bleuler, E. Primäre und sekundäre Symptome der Schizophrenie. *Zeitschzift gesellschaft für Neurologie und Psychiatrie,* 1930, *124,* 607–646.

4. Langfeldt, G. The prognosis of schizophrenia. *Acta psychiat neur Scandinavica* (Vol 31) Supplement 110, 1956.

5. American Psychiatric Association. *Diagnostic and statistical manual of mental disorders,* (3rd ed.) Washington, D.C., 1980.

6. Alanen, Y. O., Räkköläinen, V., Rasimus, R., Laakso, J., & Järvi, R. Developing the treatment of schizophrenia in a community psychiatric setting: A psychotherapeutic and family-centered approach. *Psychiatria Fennica* 1982, 101–120. Helsinki.

7. Alanen, Y. O., Räkköläinen, V., Laakso, J., Rasimus, R., & Järvi, R. Psychotherapy of schizophrenia in community psychiatry: 2-year follow-up findings and the influence of selective processes on psychotherapeutic treatments. In H. Stierlin, L. C. Wynne, & M. Wirsching (Eds.) *Psychosocial intervention in schizophrenia.* Berlin-Heidelberg: Springer, 1983.

8. Alanen, Y. O., Räkköläinen, V., Rasimus, R., & Laakso, J. Indications for the different forms of psychotherapy with new schizophrenic patients in community psychiatry. In C. Müller (Ed.) *The psychotherapy of schizophrenia*. Amsterdam-Oxford: Excerpta Medica, 1979.

9. Alanen, Y. O., Räkköläinen, V., Laakso, J., & Rasimus, R. Problems inherent in the study of psychotherapy of psychoses: Conclusions from a community psychiatric action research study. In J. S. Strauss, M. Bowers, T. W. Downey, S. Fleck, S. Jackson, & I. Levine (Eds.) *The psychotherapy of schizophrenia*, New York—London: Plenum, 1980.

10. Leff, J., & Vaughn, C. The role of maintenance therapy and relatives' expressed emotions in relapse of schizophrenia: A two-year follow-up. *British Journal of Psychiatry*, 1981, *139*, 102–104.

11. Stephens, J. H. Long-term prognosis and follow-up in schizophrenia. *Schizophrenia Bulletin* 1978, *4*, 25–47.

12. Achté, K. A. Verlauf und Prognose Schizophrener Psychosen in Helsinki. In G. W. Schimmelpenning (Ed.) *Psychiatrische Verlaufsforschung, Methoden und Ergebnisse*, Bern-Stuttgart-Wien: Huber, 1980.

13. Watt, D. C., Katz, K., & Shepherd, M. The natural history of schizophrenia: A five-year prospective follow-up of a representative sample of schizophrenics by means of a standardized clinical and social assessment. *Psychological Medicine*, 1983, *13*, 663–670.

14. von Sivers, E. En efte rundersökning av lll patienter vardade för schizofreni första gangen under aren 1961–65. With English summary. *Nordisk Psykiatrisk Tidskrift* (Vol 37) Supplement 7, 1983.

15. Winnicott, D. W. The theory of the parent-infant relationships. *International Journal of Psycho-Analysis* 1960, *41*, 585–595.

16. Salonen, S. On the technique of the psychotherapy of schizophrenia. In J. Jorstad & Ugelstad (Eds.) *Schizophrenia*, 75 Oslo: Universitetsforlaget, 1976.

17. Mosher, L. R., & Keith, S. J. Psychosocial treatment: Individual, group, family and community support approaches. *Schizophrenia Bulletin*, 1980, *6*, 10–41.

Chapter 11

THE PSYCHOLOGICAL EFFECTS OF ANTIPSYCHOTIC DRUGS

John M. Davis, M.D.
Joseph E. Comaty, M.S.
Philip G. Janicak, M.D.

This chapter will review the potential psychological effects of antipsychotic drugs on schizophrenia. It is a well established fact that antipsychotic drugs are an effective treatment for schizophrenia. Their efficacy is supported by more than 100 double-blind, randomly assigned controlled studies and by an enormous amount of clinical evidence. Since the beginning of the century, prior to the use of antipsychotic drugs, the number of schizophrenic patients who were permanent residents of state hospitals increased in proportion to the population. Immediately following the introduction of the antipsychotic drugs, the number of such hospital patients worldwide decreased dramatically. These drugs have altered how psychiatrists practice in all countries. In contrast to the preneuroleptic era, most patients are now treated on an outpatient basis with occasional exacerbations requiring hospitalization. Most of these episodic inpatient hospitalizations take place of psychiatric wards in community hospitals rather than in long-term state public hospitals. Indeed, in some countries, long-term hospital care is being completely abandoned.

ANTIPSYCHOTIC DRUGS AND THE NATURAL COURSE OF SCHIZOPHRENIA

While psychotropic drugs have had a significant and practical impact on the treatment of schizophrenia, we still are uncertain about their mechanism of action. Do antipsychotic drugs alter the natural course of schizophrenia? This is a complicated question, because before these drugs or other physical treatments were discovered there were no systematic studies of the natural course of schizophrenia, and because the cause of schizophrenia is unknown. Since we cannot make an etiologic diagnosis, we cannot define which patient has true schizophrenia and which does not. Indeed, we cannot even say whether schizophrenia is a single disease or a heterogeneous grouping of disorders. We can only approximate what the course of schizophrenia was like prior to the discovery of antipsychotic drugs. We have reviewed the clinical experience of psychiatrists with patients prior to the discovery of the neuroleptics.[1-8] We have made no attempt to separate studies done before or after electroconvulsive, insulin, or other "shock" therapy was introduced; and, hence, this data does not represent a pure picture of the natural course of untreated schizophrenia. With this caveat in mind, it appears that about 30 percent of patients diagnosed as schizophrenic at that time had a relatively good outcome and 70 percent had a very poor outcome, with most of these poor-prognosis patients spending most of their lives in a state hospital. Conversely, we have excellent evidence for the effects of antipsychotic drugs on schizophrenia in the acute phase, since most drug trials last about a month. For example, in the National Institute of Mental Health (NIMH) Collaborative Study, approximately 25 percent of the patients on placebo are substantially improved by six weeks, whereas approximately 70 percent of the patients receiving antipsychotic drugs are improved by 6 weeks.[9, 10] To arrive at these figures, we took the outcome at 6 weeks plus data from patients who either improved to such a degree that they were discharged from the hospital, otherwise terminated the study with an excellent response prior to completion, or patients who deteriorated to such an extent that drug treatment had to be introduced for ethical reasons, usually on an emergency basis. There is a striking cor-

Table 11-1. Prognosis of Schizophrenia
Before Antipsychotic Drugs

	Improvement	Same or Worse	N
Astrub	32%	68%	435
Faergeman	17%	83%	23
Rupp	34%	66%	519
Hasting	41%	59%	251
Beck	17%	83%	84
Rennie	36%	64%	456
Stalker (Review)	29%	71%	3254
Stalker	50%	50%	129
Langfeldt	23%	77%	132
TOTAL	32%	68%	5283

respondence between the short-term outcome on placebo and the long-term outcome prior to the discovery of antipsychotic drugs. That is, in both situations about 25 percent of schizophrenics improved in a 6 week period. It might be anticipated that a few more patients would improve at a somewhat slower time course so that the 25 percent at 6 weeks could become 30 percent in several years.

If an episode of schizophrenia is untreated and follows a natural course, is there a deterioration process? Does an interruption of this process with treatment reverse the deterioration? There is little evidence relevant to this other than a gross comparison of the natural course of the illness before or after these drugs were discovered. Because drug studies only last a month or so, this is too brief a time period to examine their effect on the natural course of schizophrenia. In order to make an estimate, it is necessary to compare patients randomly assigned to a drug-treated group versus a group which received no physical treatment, measuring ultimate prognosis. There is data from a study by May and his coworkers (1976) which is relevant.[11, 12] In this study, newly admitted schizophrenics were randomly assigned to five groups: No specific treatment, psychotherapy with no drugs, drug therapy, drug therapy plus psychotherapy, and ECT. Patients remained in Phase I of the study 6 months to 1 year. The authors felt that eventually, if a patient did not recover without drugs, drugs should be added. In other words, after 6 months to a year, non-drug treated patients could receive drugs. Patients receiving physical treatments had a short-term outcome far superior to that of those receiving either no specific treatment or psychotherapy alone. However, at the termination of the initial part of the study (Phase I), all patients could then receive drugs. Eventually, every patient recovered. We note parenthetically that principally good-prognosis, first-admission patients were included in the study. Patients underwent a 3-to-5 year follow-up period. During this time, all patients could receive any indicated treatment. In other words, treatment was not controlled at this time point. At follow-up, the authors measured days in hospital after first-release as an index of how well the patients were doing. This roughly equates a few long hospitalizations against many short hospitalizations. The patients who eventually received drugs spent about a month per year in hospital in the follow-up period. Those patients who initially received a physical form of treatment spent far fewer days in hospital than those who received only psychological interventions. The latter spent about 1 3/4 times as many days in hospital during the follow-up. This is particularly striking when comparing psychotherapy alone versus drugs plus psychotherapy. Those receiving psychotherapy alone spent almost twice the number of days in the hospital as those receiving drugs plus psychotherapy.

It appears that interruption of an acute episode with a somatic form of treatment results in a much better outcome over the next 3 years regardless of other treatments the patient may engage in during the follow-up period. We do not know the mechanism, but it appears that drugs have quite a substantial effect on the natural history of schizophrenia. It appears that if a patient becomes psychotic and is allowed to remain psychotic, 70 percent or so of such patients will remain sick or become sicker than they were when they presented for admission. If you allow the patients to remain psychotic for some extended period of time, these patients do much less well than if you interrupted early on with the drug form or this somatic form of treatment. It would therefore seem prudent to interrupt the psychotic process with drug treatment.

What then is the prognosis of schizophrenia? This is a slightly different question than, "If you did not initially treat, what is the natural course of a schizophrenic episode?" After drug treatment, if a reasonably good recovery is attained, the patient is able to return home. There have been a number of studies where recovered patients have been placed on placebo, as a control group for studies of maintenance antipsychotic medication.[13] At the beginning of the study, 100 percent of patients were not yet relapsed, and the number of patients "not yet relapsed" decreased with time as patients relapsed. To me, as a clinical pharmacologist, this appeared to be similar to a half-life curve. This suggested to me that one could think about the kinetics of relapse. If the rate at which patients relapsed is constant, most schizophrenic patients would have periodicity of their illnesses; for example, they would relapse every 2 to 3 years, and one would expect the relapse rate to be low, initially rising to a peak at 1 to 2 years and then declining. On the other hand, if there was some supersensitivity phenomena, patients might be at high risk for relapse the first several months following discontinuance of drugs, and then this would drop to a lower rate. We examined the data from several large double-blind controlled studies and fit the data to a model, possibly a constant relapse rate over time, which is the simplest mathematical model. There is a phenomena involving half-life of drug in the body or relapse or in an opposite direction compound interest and inflation. For example, if the relapse rate is 10 percent per month and you start a study with 100 patients not at relapse, then in the first month 10 percent, or 10, relapsed, leaving 90 patients. In the next month, 10 percent of 90, or 9, patients relapsed, leaving 81 patients. Then in the following month, 10 percent of 81, or 8 patients relapsed, leaving 72 percent of patients still in the study. The curvature in such plots accounts for this interest-on-interest phenomena. The data in these three collaborative studies[14-17] suggest that a relapse rate of schizophrenia is constant over time at 10 to 15 percent per month. There is no evidence from these studies that there was a marked increase in the relapse rate in the first month or two. This does not necessarily mean that there may not be some supersensitive phenomena in the weeks or months following drug discontinuance. It is only that this is insufficient to produce a major alteration in relapse rate in studies which did not specifically focus on such phenomenon.

BIOLOGICAL MECHANISM OF ACTION OF THE ANTIPSYCHOTIC DRUGS

The biological mechanism of action of the antipsychotics is known beyond a reasonable doubt. These drugs benefit the schizophrenic disorder by blocking the dopamine D-2 receptors in the brain and thus interfere with dopaminergic transmission. This is established by the striking correlation between the potency of blocking dopamine receptors and clinical potency of dose[18-20] as well as by the striking correlation between both these variables and a variety of behavioral tests for dopaminergic action or other biochemical changes produced by these drugs consequent to decreased dopaminergic transmission.[18-20] In addition, Johnstone, Crow and their coworkers[21] have shown that the isomer which has the property of blocking dopamine receptors is the isomer that is clinically active. Carlson[22] and his coworkers have shown that if dopamine synthesis is reduced by the administration of alpha-methyl-p-tyrosine, the dose of antipsychotic drug necessary for optimal clinical efficacy is consequently reduced. What is unknown, however, is what dopamine blockade has to do with schizophrenia, since the cause of schizophrenia still remains undiscovered. There is some evidence that schizophrenics may have either high levels of brain dopamine or supersensitive dopamine receptors. El Youseph Janowsky and Davis[23] administered methylphenidate to schizophrenic patients and observed that the psychosis was markedly intensified. This dose of methylphenidate usually causes only mild euphoria in normal individuals. Furthermore, after the psychotic episode was over (whether by spontaneous remission or drug treatment), methylphenidate no longer activated psychotic symptoms.[24] If the recovering schizophrenic patients have their maintenance drugs terminated and then a test-dose of psychomotor stimulant is administered, patients who show the transitory psychomotor stimulant-induced psychosis are those who are at greatest risk for early relapse. This finding is quite consistent with the state-dependency of the psychomotor-induced worsening of psychosis observed by Janowsky and Davis.[23] We would further note that a variety of drugs can often produce a paranoid psychosis and hallucinations as a side effect when given to parkinsonian patients. These include L-dopa (which is converted to dopamine); amantadine (which has dopaminergic and anticholinergic properties), bromocriptine; and a wide variety of direct dopamine agonists (e.g., amphetamine, Ritalin); and a variety of psychomotor stimulants, such as cocaine, which is a potent blocker of dopamine reuptake. The duration of amphetamine-induced psychosis corresponds to the length of time the drug remains in the body. In addition, the cocaine-induced paranoia often dissipates within an hour after ingestion is stopped, corresponding to the rapid half-life of cocaine. Thus, while there is evidence that implicates dopamine in psychosis, the paranoid psychosis induced by drugs is not identical to schizophrenia. What we know is that the antipsychotic action of neuroleptics is due to their dopamine-receptor blocking effects. Since drugs that are dopaminergic in some sense can cause a type of psychosis, although an imperfect model, this further strengthens the relevance of dopamine to psychosis. In summary, since we do not know the cause of schizophrenia, we do not know exactly how dopamine blockade relates to the causative factors of schizophrenia, or how it produces an alleviation of that disorder.

THE PSYCHOLOGICAL MECHANISM OF ACTION OF ANTIPSYCHOTIC DRUGS

We collated data from a wide variety of rating-scale studies used to quantitate drug-induced improvement.[9, 26] Drug-induced changes are seen for virtually all the symptomatic abnormalities of schizophrenic patients, and the pattern of improvement suggests that all symptoms thought to be psychotic in general are seen in schizophrenia and reduced by neuroleptics.[9, 25]

Schizophrenia is also characterized by a marked disturbance of thought. It is important to make the distinction between disturbance of thought as measured by testing for thought disorder as opposed to a psychiatrist's rating of thought disorder based on observation of such manifestations as hallucinations or delusions. We want to emphasize the distinction between thought disorder as defined and operationally measured with a variety of conceptual models versus "crazy behavior or thoughts" in a more general sense. We worked with observations of Phil Holzman and Steve Hurt to study the effects of antipsychotic drugs on thought disorder.[26] Holzman had devised a method for measuring thought disorder involving the administration of standard stimuli provided by psychological tests. The schizophrenic's responses to these stimuli were recorded, then evaluated for the presence or absence of thought disorder and, if present, rated in its severity. This instrument evaluated a wide variety of thought disorders. In essence, a schizophrenic's thoughts were elicited to a common stimuli, and then the psychologists counted the number of disturbed thoughts. When we plotted the rate of improvement in thought disorder and the rate of improvement of the schizophrenia, we found that antipsychotic drugs produced the same rate of alleviation of thought disorder as the rate of alleviation of symptoms of schizophrenia. We concluded that antipsychotic drugs benefit thought disorder with a similar time course as they benefit the other symptoms of schizophrenia.

ANTIPSYCHOTIC DRUGS AND NEGATIVE SYMPTOMS

Elsewhere in this volume, Dr. Crow has discussed the importance of the conceptual division of schizophrenic symptoms into negative and positive symptoms.[27] We investigated several aspects of the classification of symptoms into positive and negative symptoms. One of our coworkers, Dr. Richard Lewine, reviewed the individual items assessed by the Inpatient Multidimensional Psychiatric Scale—a 78-item rating scale filled out on the basis of clinical interviews lasting approximately 1 hour. Each item was rated on a scale of 1 to 9. For this purpose, Dr.

Lewine selected items representing two theoretical views of negative symptoms. In collaboration with our statistician, Dr. Robert Gibbons, we analyzed the data from this efficacy study by a relatively new statistical methodology which characterized the N-dimensional latent distribution of the ratings. They were log-transferred for a better approximation of a normal distribution. A maximal-likelihood-factor analysis was then performed to determine the latent distribution of the symptoms.

Using the computer program EFAP, we estimated 1 to 5 dimensional models for these data. We then determined which model yielded the fewest factors and used a chi-square statistic indicating a good fit for the data. We performed a confirmatory factor analysis using LISREL. The symptoms included in the analysis were slowed speech, irrelevant speech, incoherent speech, wandering speech, apathy toward treatment, fixed facial expression, slow movements, thought blocking, apathy toward environment, poverty of speech, and inappropriate affect. A three-factor model fit the data. One-factor and two-factor models were massively discrepant with the data. If negative symptoms were a unified cluster of symptoms, then a one-dimensional model should fit the data. This was clearly not the case. The first factor we labelled "apathy," since it had high loadings on the two apathy items. The second factor we labelled "retardation," which had high loadings on slow speech, slow movements, and poverty of speech. The third factor we labelled "Bleulerian symptoms," since it had high loadings on irrelevant speech, incoherent speech, wandering speech, and inappropriate affect. The score on each item loading on the "apathy" factor or on the "retardation" factor or on the Bleulerian" factor can be weighted and combined into a numerical score reflecting the latent dimension described by these factors.

We then plotted a frequency distribution for each of these scores. If the patient's scores were normally distributed on this scale, one might expect the frequency distribution to be a Gaussian normal distribution, with the average schizophrenic showing a moderate amount of disturbance and a few patients showing either little or a great deal of disturbance. This is not the case. For each of these three variables, the frequency distribution is bimodal. For the apathy factor, 77 percent of the subjects have a mean of 2.5 on this dimension, and 24 percent of the subjects have a mean of 5.5. There are thus two peaks, one approximately double the intensity of the other. For the retardation factor, 75 percent of the subjects have a mean of 2.0, and 25 percent of the subjects have a mean of 5.6. For the Bleulerian factor, 72 percent of the subjects have a mean of 1.8, and 28 percent of the subjects have a mean of 4.4.

It would seem that for each of these three variables, the patients could be characterized as either having or not having the symptom complex. It appears that about 25 percent of the subjects are characterized as apathetic, about 25 percent as retarded, and about 25 percent as having the Bleulerian-negative symptoms: i.e., irrelevant, incoherent, wandering speech and inappropriate affect. Thus, 25 percent of the patients have each of the three types of negative symptoms. If negative symptoms were unified concepts, you would expect that those patients who are apathetic are also retarded as well as have the Bleulerian symptoms. The fact that these variables have bimodal frequency histograms suggests that these variables are not continuously distributed in a Gaussian normal distribution, but that the high group consists of patients who have the syndrome and those who are in the low subgroup are those who do not have the syndrome. Thus there is a subgroup of apathetic schizophrenics, a subgroup of retarded schizophrenics, and a subgroup of "Bleulerian" (irrelevant speech, flat affect, etc.) schizophrenics. If negative symptoms was, indeed, a subdivision of schizophrenia, then if a patient is in the high subgroup for one factor, he should be in the high subgroups for the other two factors. This is not the case. There is a rare patient who has both apathy and the Bleulerian cluster, but this is no more than would be expected by chance (chi-square = 1.49; not statistically significant). Similarly, it is a relatively rare patient who has both retardation and the Bleulerian-negative symptoms. (p = .04).

This is in a direction that suggests that retardation is seen less frequently with Bleulerian negative symptoms than expected by chance alone. Ten percent of patients have retardation but do not have apathy; 10 percent have apathy but not retardation; 10 percent have both and 70 percent neither. This is a significant statistical association. However, the association that two out of three have one symptom cluster but not the other is not statistically significant, so that there is not a one to one correlation between apathy and retardation. When patients receiving the antipsychotic drugs are compared to those who received placebo, there are clearly statistical improvements in drug versus placebo on all three negative-symptom factors. However, the degree of improvement, that is the drug-placebo difference, is substantially greater for the Bleulerian-symptom factor than it is for the retardation or the apathy factor. Indeed, for the Bleulerian-symptom factor, the drug-placebo difference is in the same order of magnitude as that seen with the positive symptoms. If one were to conceptualize these results, it would be to suggest that "the Bleulerian cluster" is not a negative symptom.

COMPARATIVE EFFICACY OF DRUG TREATMENT

Although there is no way quantitatively to compare qualitatively different results, we can quantitate the drug-placebo difference of two different drugs. For example, to obtain an order-of-magnitude comparison of how well antipsychotics help schizophrenics, we compared this to streptomycin in the treatment of tuberculosis, since tuberculosis is also a chronic disease. The British Medical Research Council (MRC)[28] did a double-blind study comparing bed rest alone versus bed rest plus streptomycin. The NIMH Collaborative Study (which was reviewed above) found that about 70 percent of patients do well with treatment with antipsychotic drugs in comparison to about one-fourth of the patients with placebo. On the other hand, a little less than 50 percent of the patients on placebo markedly deteriorate, whereas only a few percent of the schizophrenics treated with antipsychotics deteriorate. In comparison, the data from the MRC Study with streptomycin found that although a little less than a third of streptomycin patients deteriorate, almost two-thirds of those on bed rest alone deteriorate. A little more than 50 percent of the patients on streptomycin have a good result, whereas less than 10 percent of those on bed rest alone have a good result.

In other words, one dichotomizes what is a continuous variable for both treatments. Seventy percent of schizophrenics, roughly speaking, do well with drug and 30 percent do relatively poorly, in contrast to 25 percent on placebo who do relatively well and 75 percent who do relatively poorly. Similarly, for streptomycin versus bed rest, 70 percent of patients do well with streptomycin and about 30 percent do relatively poorly, whereas only one-third of patients receiving bed rest alone do relatively well and two-thirds do relatively poorly. Although the percentage of patients doing relatively poorly versus relatively well is more or less comparable between these two treatments, the greatest difference in these comparisons is found in the streptomycin group who have a really good response to drug and in the schizophrenic group who deteriorate with placebo. In other words, the psychostatic action of the antipsychotics is a little more remarkable in terms of drug-placebo difference than the curative action of streptomycin.

We have previously examined the 35 controlled studies of antipsychotic drugs versus placebo for maintenance medication in 3,500 patients. Fifty-eight percent of patients on placebo experienced relapse in contrast to 16 percent of patients on drugs. There is no doubt that maintenance medication reduces the frequency of relapse. Maintenance medication can be given in two forms—an oral form and a depot intramuscular form administered every 2 weeks. We might add that there have been six studies comparing the depot medication to the oral medication for maintenance.[29-34] These results are summarized in Table 11-2. Three of these studies found fewer relapses on depot medication as compared to the oral medication, and three of the studies found little difference between the two. If we combine the data from all six studies, there is a statistically significant difference, using the Mantel-Haenszel Test,[35] showing that the use of depot medication prevented more relapses than the use of oral medication (chi-square equals 13.5, p = .0002). We would speculate that the difference among the studies may

Table 11-2.   **Percentage Differential: More Relapsed with Oral Medication**

	N	*Percent*
Crawford	29	27%
Hogarty	104	23%
Falloon et al.	41	−16%
Quitkin	34	−8%
Schooler	185	10%
Del Giudice	82	48%

Mantel-Haenszel Test   p = .0002

be explained by variable compliance with oral medication. Those studies with sick, uncooperative patients have fewer compliers than those studies with well motivated, cooperative patients; but we have no direct data to support this hypothesis. If even a few patients do not take their oral medication regularly, then when data is summated from many studies, this effect can and, apparently, here does come through.

COMPARATIVE EFFICACY OF FAMILY THERAPY

Although we have focused this review on the pharmacological effects of drugs, we would like to note that psychological factors are also important. There is a new generation of studies examining the treatment of all schizophrenics with drugs, but then varying as an experimental variable the presence or absence of psychosocial intervention. We have summarized the results from four recent studies that treated all chronic outpatient schizophrenics with maintenance antipsychotic drugs.[36–39] Patients were randomly assigned to receive drugs alone or drugs plus family therapy. When the drugs plus family therapy interaction was applied, the number of relapses remarkably decreased compared to the relapse rate in the group treated with drugs alone. Note that the efficacy of the newer treatment

**Table 11-3. Outcome of Schizophrenia Treated with
Family Therapy and Drugs Versus Drugs Alone**

	% Relapsed	
	Both	*Drugs Alone*
Golstein et al.	4%	16%
Falloon et al.	11%	50%
Hogarty*	3%	25%
Leff et al.	40%	78%
TOTAL (n = 236)	8%**	30%

*Family Therapy with or without social skills training.
**Average computed by summing results on number of subjects in each
study.

(drugs plus family therapy) measured against the older standard treatment (drugs alone) shows about a three to one efficacy
factor. This is comparable to the efficacy factor of antipsychotic
drugs versus placebo or of streptomycin in comparison to bed
rest alone.

REFERENCES

1. Astrup, C., Fossum, A., & Holmboe, R. *Prognosis in functional psychoses*. Springfield, Ill.: Charles C. Thomas, 1962.
2. Beck, M.N. Twenty-five and thirty-five year follow-up of first admissions to mental hospitals. *Canadian Psychiatric Association
   Journal, 13*, 1968: 219–229.
3. Faergeman, P.M. *Psychogenic psychoses*. London: Butterworth, 1963.
4. Hastings, D.W. Follow-up results in psychiatric illness. *American
   Journal of Psychiatry*, 1958, *114*, 1–11.
5. Langfeldt, G. Schizophrenia: Diagnosis and prognosis. *Behavioral
   Science*, 1969, *14*, 173–182.
6. Rennie, T.A.C. Follow-up study of five-hundred patients with
   schizophrenia admitted to the hospital from 1913 to 1923. *Archives of Neurological Psychiatry*, 1939, *42*, 877–891.

7. Rupp, C., & Fletcher, E. A five- to ten-year follow-up study of 641 schizophrenic cases. *American Journal of Psychiatry*, 1939, *96*, 877–888.

8. Stalker, H. Prognosis in schizophrenia. *Journal of Mental Science*, 1939, *85*, 1224–1240.

9. Cole, J.O., Goldberg, S.C., & Davis, J.M. Drugs in the treatment of psychosis: Controlled studies. In P. Solomon, (Ed.), *Psychiatric drugs*. New York: Grune & Stratton, 1966.

10. Cole, J.O., Goldberg, S.C. & Klerman, J. Phenothiazine treatment in acute schizophrenia. Effectiveness. *Archives of General Psychiatry*, 1964, *10*, 246–261.

11. May, P.R.A., Tuma, A.H., & Dixon, W.J. Schizophrenia: A follow-up study of results of treatments. I Design and other problems. *Archives of General Psychiatry*, 1976, *33*, 474–480.

12. May, P.R.A., Tuma, A.H., Yale, C., Potepan, P., & Dixon, W.J. Schizophrenia: A follow-up study of results of treatment. II. Hospital stay over two to five years. *Archives of General Psychiatry*, 1976, *33*, 481–486.

13. Davis, J.M. Overview: Maintenance therapy in psychiatry: I. Schizophrenia, *American Journal of Psychiatry*, 1975, *132*, 1237–1245.

14. Caffey, E.M., Diamond, L.S., Frank, T.V., Grasberger, J.C., Herman, L., Klett, C.J., & Rothstein, D. Discontinuation or reduction of chemotherapy in chronic schizophrenics. *Journal of Chronic Disease*, 1964, *17*, 347–358.

15. Hogarty, G.E., & Goldberg, S.C. Drugs and sociotherapy in the aftercare of schizophrenic patients. One-year relapse rates. *Archives of General Psychiatry*, 1973, *28*, 54–64.

16. Hogarty, G.E. & Ulrich, R.F. Temporal effects of drug and placebo in delaying relapse in schizophrenic outpatients. *Archives of General Psychiatry*, 1977, *34*, 297–301.

17. Hogarty, G.E., Goldberg, S.C., Schooler, N.R., & Ulrich, R.F. Drugs and sociotherapy in the aftercare of schizophrenic patients. *Archives of General Psychiatry*, 1974, *31*, 603–608.

18. Seeman, P., Lee, T., Chau-Wong, M., & Wong, K. Antipsychotic drug doses and neuroleptic/dopamine receptors. *Nature*, 1976, *261*, 717–719.

19. Snyder, S.H., Creese, I., & Burt, D.R. The brain's dopamine re-

ceptor: Labelling with ³H-dopamine and ³H-haloperidol. *Communications in Psychopharmacology*, 1975, *1*, 663–673.

20. Horn, A.S., & Snyder, S.H. Chlorpromazine and dopamine: Conformational similarities that correlate with the antischizophrenic activity of phenothiazine drugs. *Proceedings of the Academy of Science*, 1971, *65*, 2325.

21. Johnstone, E.C., Crow, T.J., Frith, C.D., Carney, M.W.P., & Price, J.S. Mechanism of the antipsychotic effect in the treatment of acute schizophrenia. *Lancet*, 1978, *1*, 848.

22. Carlson, A. Antipsychotic drugs, neurotransmitters, and schizophrenia. *American Journal of Psychiatry*, 1978, *135*, 164.

23. Janowsky, D.S., El-Yousef, M.K., Davis, J.M., & Sekerke, H.J. Provocation of schizophrenic symptoms by intravenous administration of methylphenidate. *Archives of General Psychiatry*, 1973, *28*, 185–191.

24. Angrist, B., & VanKammen, D.P. CNS stimulants as tools in the study of schizophrenia. *Trends in Neuroscience*, 1984, *8*, 388–390.

25. Davis, J.M., Schaffer, C.B., Killian, G.A., Kinard, C., & Chan, C. Important issues in the drug treatment of schizophrenia. *Schizophrenia Bulletin*, 1980, *6*, 70–87.

26. Hurt, S.W., Holzman, P.S., & Davis, J.M. Thought disorder. *Archives of General Psychiatry*, 1981, *40*, 1281.

27. Gibbons, R.D., Lewine, R.R.J., Davis, J.M., Schooler, N.R., & Cole, J.O. An empirical test of a Kraepelinian vs. a Bleulerian view of negative symptoms. *Schizophrenia Bulletin*, 1985, *11 (3)*, 390–396.

28. Medical Research Council. Streptomycin treatment of pulmonary tuberculosis. A Medical Research Council investigation. *British Medical Journal*, October 30, 1948, 769–782.

29. Del Guidice, J., Clark, W.G., & Gocka, E.F. Prevention of recidivism of schizophrenics treated with fluphenazine enanthate. *Psychosomatics*, 1975, *16*, 32–36.

30. Crawford, R., & Forrest, A. Controlled trial of depot fluphenazine in outpatient schizophrenics. *British Journal of Psychiatry*, 1974, *124*, 385–391.

31. Falloon, I., Watt, D.C. & Shepherd, M. A comparative controlled trial of pimozide and fluphenazine decanoate in the continuation therapy of schizophrenia. *Psychological Medicine*, 1978, *8*, 59–70.

32. Hogarty, G.E., Schooler, N.R., Ulrich, R., Mussare, F., Ferro, P., & Herron, E. Fluphenazine and social therapy in the aftercare of schizophrenic patients: Relapse analyses of a two-year controlled study of fluphenazine decanoate and fluphenazine hydrochloride. *Archives of General Psychiatry*, 1979, *36*, 1283–1294.
33. Schooler, N.R., Levine, J., & Severe, J.B. Depot fluphenazine in the prevention of relapse in schizophrenia: Evaluation of a treatment regimen. *Psychopharmacology Bulletin*, 1978, *15*, 44.
34. Quitkin, F., Rifkin, A., Kane, J., Ramos-Loren, J.R. & Klein, D.F. Long-acting oral vs injectable antipyschotic drugs in schizophrenia. *Archives of General Psychiatry*, 1978, *35*, 889–892.
35. Mantel, N., & Haenszel, W. Statistical aspects of the analysis of data from retrospective studies of disease. *Journal of the National Cancer Institute*, 1959, *22*, 719–748.
36. Goldstein, M.J., Rodnick, E., Evans, J., May, P., & Steinberg, M. Drug and family in the aftercare of acute schizophrenics. *Archives of General Psychiatry*, 1978, *35*, 1169–1177.
37. Leff, J., Kuipers, L., Berkowitz, R., et al. A controlled trial of social intervention in the families of schizophrenic patients. *British Journal of Psychiatry*, 1982, *141*, 121–134.
38. Hogarty, G.E. Depot neuroleptics: The relevance of pschosocial factors—A United States perspective. *Journal of Clinical Psychiatry*, 1984, *45*, 36–42.
39. Falloon, I. R. H., Boyd, J. L., McGill, C. W. et al. Family management in the prevention of exacerbations of schizophrenia: A controlled study. *New England Journal of Medicine* 1982, *306*, 1437–1440.

Chapter 12

NALOXONE IN SCHIZOPHRENIC HALLUCINATIONS

Yiannis G. Papakostas, M.D.

Naloxone administration in schizophrenia represents a common clinical strategy to test the hypothesis of endogenous opioid peptides' involvement in the pathophysiology of this disorder.[1-5] Within this context auditory hallucinations have been the target symptom on which the effect of naloxone has been most frequently tested.[6]

During a study that was conducted at the Northport Veteran's Hospital in New York, the effect of naloxone was examined in 5 schizophrenic male patients with auditory hallucinations. Auditory hallucinations representing the target symptom of treatment with naloxone should be present as a prominent symptom and for a minimum of two occurrences per hour. Having established such a strict inclusion criterion, it is not surprising that from a large hospital population we were able to find only five patients fitting those requirements. All five patients were on neuroleptics and other psychotropic drugs long before initiation of this study. Their pharmaceutical status was kept unchanged throughout the course of this study.

Initially, an open study was conducted: During this each patient received six different doses of naloxone IV as a bolus (0.4, 1.2, 4.0, 10, 15, and 30 mg) at a frequency of no more than two trials a week. Whenever it was believed that a particular dose

Table 12-1. Experiences with Naloxone
as Antihallucinogen

Subject	Open Trial (Naloxone in mg, IV)						Double-Blind Crossover Trial Naloxone (Nal) vs Placebo (Pl)		
								Session	
	0.4	1.2	4.0	10.	15.	30.	Dose	First	Second
1	−	−	+	−	−	−	4.0	−	+ (PL)
2	−	−	−	+	−	−	10.	+ (Nal)	−
3	−	+	−	−	−	−	4.0	−	−
4	−	±	−	±	−	−	10.	−	−
5	−	−	−	−	−	−	No trial		

+ Effect
− No Effect

elicited symptoms reduction, this dose was then reexamined under double-blind conditions matched against placebo. The patients were rated with four behavioral scales—including one specifically designed for assessment of hallucinations—before, as well as l/2, 1, 2, 3, and 6 hours after naloxone administration.

In the open trial, subject 1 had a positive response (reduction of hallucinations) with the 4.0 mg naloxone dose. During the double-blind trial with the same dose a positive response was obtained. However, upon breaking the code it was found that this response was elicited by the placebo.

Subject 2 had a positive response with the dose of 10 mg and again another positive response during the double-blind trial which turned out to be elicited by naloxone.

Subject 3 and 4 responded favorably during the open trial but no response was elicited during the double-blind trial.

No double-blind trial was conducted on the subject 5 since no positive response was noticed during the open (dose-finding) study (Table 12-l).

Our findings are inconclusive since a definite naloxone effect on schizophrenic hallucinations was not obtained. Muesser and Dysken[6] in their systematic review of the literature reported a clear, if only temporary, general antipsychotic effect on some patients. However there is no concluded remark as far as the antihallucinatory effect of naloxone is concerned. Verhoeven et al.[7] in their review estimated that about one-fourth of the schizophrenic patients had a temporary reduction of auditory hallucinations. It is therefore possible that a certain number of patients may respond favorably to naloxone, as was the case with our patient.

Identification of these "responders" and repeated double-blind trials with naloxone may be necessary for future studies on the effect of naloxone on schizophrenic hallucinations.

REFERENCES

1. Gunne, L.M., Lindström, L., Terenius, L. Naloxone-induced reversal of schizophrenic hallucinations. *Journal of Neural Transmission*, 1977, *40*, 13–19.
2. Volavka, J., Mallya, A., Baig, S., et al. Naloxone in chronic schizophrenia *Science*, 1977, *196*, 1277–1228.
3. Emrich, H.M., Cording, C., Piree, S., et al. Indication of an antipsychotic action of the opiate antagonist naloxone, *Pharmakipsychiatrie/Neyro-psychopharmakologie*, 1977, *10*, 265–270.
4. Davis, G.C., Bunney, W.E. Jr., De-Fraites, E.G., et al. Intravenous naloxone adminstration in schizophrenia and affective disorders. *Science*, 1977, *197*, 74–77.
5. Watson, S.J., Berger, P.A., Akil, H., et al. Effects of naloxone in schizophrenia: Reduction in hallucinations in a subpopulation of subjects. *Science*, 1978, *201*, 73–76.
6. Mueser, K.T., Dysken, M.W. Narcotic antagonists in schizophrenia: A methodological review. *Schizophrenia Bulletin*, 1983, 9/2, 213–225.
7. Verhoeven, W.M.A., van Prag, H.M., van Ree, J.M. Repeated naloxone administration in schizophrenia. *Psychiatry Research*, 1984, *12*, 297–312.

Chapter 13

EFFECTS OF ECT ON NOCTURNAL PROLACTIN SECRETION IN SCHIZOPHRENICS

Preliminary Observations

Constantin R. Soldatos, M.D.,
Joanne D. Bergiannaki, M.D.,
Paul N. Sakkas, M.D.,
John Kibouris, M.D., Georgia Sakellariou, M.D.,
and Costas N. Stefanis, M.D.

An immediate and short-lasting increase in plasma prolactin (PRL) concentrations has been previously reported as a characteristic effect of electroconvulsive therapy (ECT)[1] in both depressed[2-5] and schizophrenic patients,[6] as well as of electroconvulsive shock (ECS) in animal experiments.[7] Previous studies[1, 2, 8] however, were limited to the daytime only, i.e. have shown an increase of plasma PRL levels 5 minutes to 1 hour following ECT, and a subsequent return to pretreatment levels.[3] Since PRL normally peaks at night,[9, 10] we focused on the effects of ECT on nocturnal PRL secretion.

The aim of this study was to investigate the effect of a single ECT on the nocturnal plasma PRL concentrations in schizophrenic patients, as well as its possible relation to the type of psychopathology of the patients and the therapeutic outcome of a series of 8—12 ECTs.

MATERIAL AND METHODS

Seven male psychiatric inpatients (mean age 27.14 years, range 18 to 43) free of any endocrine or other medical disorder were studied. In each case the diagnosis of a schizophrenic disorder was based on DSM III criteria and was established independently by two psychiatrists. The patients had not taken any medication for at least 15 days prior to entering the study, except for three who took a benzodiazepine (lorazepam 2.5 mg/daily P.O. in one case, and diazepam 20 mg/daily P.O. in two cases) at a fixed regimen throughout the study.

All patients were premedicated one-half hour prior to ECT with atropine sulfate 1 mg i.m. and immediately before the application of ECT with 50 mg pentothal sodium i.v. In each case, a bilateral ECT at about 10 a.m. produced generalized convulsions of a 30–35 sec. duration. Following this first session, each patient had a series of ECTs with a frequency of application of 2–3 per week to a total of 8–12 sessions and a cumulative duration of convulsions at least 240 sec. Until termination of the series each patient was not allowed any additional treatment modality.

Blood was sampled hourly for 12 consecutive hours starting at 9 p.m. on 2 nights (the night before and the night after the first ECT). Each hourly sample was collected using an antecubital intravenous needle attached to a continuous blood withdrawal pump (CORMED ML 6-3).[11] It was then centrifuged and the serum was stored in -20°C until the hormonal determination, which was accomplished at the same time for all the samples through a radioimmunoassay method with reagents from BIODATA S.p.A. standardized with the IRP of human PRL for immunoassay (75/504). The values for PRL plasma levels were expressed in milli-international units per milliliter (mIU/ml).

Except for the unavoidable postconvulsive sleep of relatively short duration (in no case more than 1 hour), the patients were not allowed to sleep until 10 p.m., at which time they went to bed until 6 a.m. the next day. In three cases, sleep was recorded in the sleep laboratory; for the remaining four, it was closely monitored through observations by the nursing staff.

Overall psychopathology was evaluated in each case utilizing BPRS[12] at two time points: on baseline and after completion of the series of ECTs. Data were analysed using the paired t-test.

RESULTS

For the total sample of our seven patients the average value of nocturnal PRL secretion showed only a very slight increase (0.42 ± 0.90, pre-ECT vs. 0.48 ± 0.30, post-ECT; $p < 0.1$). Nevertheless, when observing individual patient values, we were able to discriminate between two groups: group A including three cases with a clear-cut increase (0.32 ± 0.06 vs 0.43 ± 0.13, $p < 0.01$) and group B which included the remaining four cases with no significant increase (0.49 ± 0.14 vs 0.52 ± 0.12 N.S.); actually, in group B there was one case in which nocturnal PRL showed significant decrease (0.46 ± 0.12 vs 0.31 ± 0.06, $p < 0.01$).

The two groups (Table) did not differ in terms of the level of their overall psychopathology, as expressed by the total BPRS score (55.33 ± 4.16 for group A vs 56.00 ± 9.05 for group B, N.S.). They did differ, however, in terms of specific clusters of BPRS items as well as duration of illness. Thus, as shown on the Table, group A scored higher in items which are characteristic of "positive" schizophrenic symptomatology (hallucinatory behavior, grandiosity, suspiciousness, hostility, tension, anxiety) and lower in items typical for symptomatology of the "negative" type (emotional withdrawal, blunted affect, conceptual disorganization and motor retardation). Further, the patients in group A had a shorter duration of illness (1.5 ± 0.5 vs 12.8 ± 5.0 years).

Depending on the presence or absence of an increase in nocturnal PRL secretion following the first ECT, our patients showed a differential therapeutic response after completion of

Table 13-1.   Treatment Outcome of ECT as a Function of Its Initial Effect on Nocturnal Prolactin

	Group A ● (N=3)		Group B ■ (N=4)	
	Baseline	*After series of ECTs*	*Baseline*	*After series of ECTs*
BPRS score Total	55.3±4.1	38.3±1.5**	56.0±9.0	52.7±10.6
Positive symptoms	26.3±0.5	16.0±2.6*	16.5±4.0	15.2±3.2
Negative symptoms	14.0±3.6	9.0±4.0*	20.0±3.5	19.7±3.7
Duration of illness (yrs)	1.5±0.5		12,8±5,0	

● Group A: increase in nocturnal PRL following the first ECT
■ Group B: no increase in nocturnal PRL following the first ECT
* $p<0.05$
** $p<0.01$

a series of ECTs (Table). Thus, for group A there was a significant decrease in the overall BPRS score, both in terms of "positive" as well as "negative" clusters of items. Patients in group B, on the other hand, did not show any considerable change in psychopathology after the termination of their ECTs, as reflected in the overall BPRS score and the scores in both the "positive" and the "negative" items. It is noteworthy that the sole patient who showed a significant decrease of nocturnal PRL had all the trends observed in group B more pronounced, i.e. more intense "negative" symptomatology and an unfavorable treatment outcome.

DISCUSSION

Our data show that the effects of ECT on PRL levels are less uniform for the first post-ECT night than for the period of a few minutes immediately following the convulsions. Thus, although an increase in PRL has been almost invariably observed immediately following the ECT[1, 6] the nocturnal PRL levels have been increased by ECT in some of our patients but not in others. Further, patients showing a post-ECT increase in nocturnal PRL (group A) had more florid schizophrenic symptoms and responded positively to a series of ECTs, whereas patients who did not show an ECT-induced increase in nocturnal PRL (group B) had more symptoms of a "defect" schizophrenic state and had a poorer therapeutic outcome.

Some forms of schizophrenic illness are associated with central dopaminergic hyperactivity[13–16] which is reflected indirectly to plasma PRL levels.[17–20] According to Crow,[21] Type I schizophrenic syndrome (characterized by positive symptoms) is in some way associated with a change in dopaminergic transmission,[22] while type II schizophrenic syndrome (characterized by negative symptoms) is unrelated to dopaminergic transmission.[21] Further, patients with positive schizophrenic symptoms respond more favorably to ECT[23] as well as to treatment with neuroleptic drugs,[21] whose antipsychotic activity is directly related to their potency in inhibiting the dopaminergic system.[24]

The increase in nocturnal PRL secretion in our group A

patients, who had symptoms similar to those of type I schizo-phrenic syndrome[21] is probably related to a delayed inhibitory effect of ECT on the dopaminergic system or to a more complex sequence of neurochemical changes, which follow the acute inhibition of dopaminergic neurons and affect sleep-related mechanisms of PRL secretion. As reflected in our results, this more profound antidopaminergic effect of ECT is most likely related to the therapeutic efficacy of the series of ECTs.

In contrast to the immediate PRL response to ECT, which is more general, the response of nocturnal PRL secretion appears to be more specific and could serve as an early prognostic index of the effectiveness of a series of ECTs in schizophrenia. To confirm and further evaluate these preliminary observations, more extensive investigations are needed, including a greater number of schizophrenic patients, studied for an entire 24-hour period. Also, the effects of ECT on 24-hour PRL secretion need to be studied following a complete series of ECTs.

REFERENCES

1. Arató, M., Erdós, A., Kurcz, M., Vermes, I., & Fekete, M. Studies on the prolactin response induced by eletroconvulsive therapy in schizophrenics. *Acta psychiatrica scandavica*. 1980, *61*, 239–244.
2. Ohman, R., Balldin, J., Walinder, J., & Wallin, L. Prolactin response to electroconvulsive therapy. *Lancet*, 1976, *i*, 936–937.
3. O'Dea, J.P.K., Gould, D.B.Sc., Hallberg, M., & Wieland, R.G. Prolactin changes during electroconvulsive therapy. *American Journal of Psychiatry*, 1978, *135*, 5, 609–611.
4. Deakin, J.F.W., Ferrier, I.N., Crow, T.J., Johnstone, E.E., & Lawter, P. Effects of ECT on pituitary hormone release: Relationship to seizure, clinical variables and outcome. *British Journal of Psychiatry*, 1983, *143*, 618–624.
5. Linnoila, M., Litovitz, G., Scheinin, M., Chang, M.D., & Gutler, N.R. Effects of electroconvulsive treatment on monoamine metabolites, growth hormone, and prolactin in plasma. *Biological Psychiatry*, 1984, *19*, 1, 79–83.
6. Meco, G., Casacchia, M., Carchedi, F., Falaschi, P., Rocco, A., &

Frajese, G. Prolactin response to repeated electroconvulsive therapy in acute schizophrenia. *Lancet*, 1978, *i*, 999.

7. Essman, W.B. Antidepressant action of electroconvulsive therapy. *Lancet*, 1978, *i*, 935.

8. Whalley, L.J., Dick, H., Watts, A.G., Christie, J.E., Rosie, R., Levy, G., Sheward, W.J., & Fink G. Immediate increases in plasma prolactin and neurophysin but not other hormones after electroconvulsive therapy. *Lancet*, 1982, *i*, 1064–1065.

9. Sassin, J.F., Frantz, A.G., Kapen, S., et al. The nocturnal rise of human prolactin is dependent on sleep. *Journal of Clinical Endocrinology and Metabolism*, 1973, *37*, 436–440.

10. Weitzman, E.D., Boyar, R.M., Kapen, S., & Hellman, L. The relationship of sleep and sleep stages to neuroendocrine secretion and biological rhythms in man. *Recent Progress Hormonal Research*, 1975, *31*, 399–441.

11. Kowarski, A., Thomspon, R.G., Migeon, C.J., & Blizzard, R.M. Determination of integrated plasma concentrations and true secretion rates of human growth hormone. *Journal of Clinical Endocrinology and Metabolism*, 1971, *32*, 356.

12. Overall, J.E. The Brief Psychiatric Rating Scale in psychopharmacology research in psychological measurements. In *Psychopharmacology, Modern Problems in Pharmacopsychiatry*, 7, pp. 67–78 P. Pichot (Ed.), Paris/Basel:Karger, 1974.

13. Horn, A.S., Snyder, S.H. Chlorpromazine and dopamine: Conformational similarities that correlate with the antischizophrenic activity of phenothiazine drugs. *Proceedings National Academy Science*, U.S.A., 1971, *68*, 2325–2328.

14. Randrup, A., & Munkvard, I. Evidence indicating an association between schizophrenia and dopaminergic hyperactivity in the brain. *Orthomollecular Psychiatry*, 1972, *1*, 2–7.

15. Friedhoff, A.J. & Alpert, M. A dopaminergic-cholinergic mechanism in production of psychotic symptoms. *Biological Psychiatry*, 1973, *6*, 165–169.

16. Matthysse, S. Antipsychotic drug actions: A clue to the neuropathology of schizophrenia? *Federation Proceedings*, 1973, *32*, 200–205.

17. Meltzer, H.Y., Sachar, E.J. & Frantz, A.G. Serum prolactin levels in unmedicated schizophrenic patients. *Archives General Psychiatry*, 1974, *31*, 564–569.

18. Meites, J. Catecholamines and prolactin secretion. In Costa, E., & G.L. Gessa (Eds.) *Advances in biochemical psychopharmacology, (Vol. 16)*. New York: Raven Press, 1977.
19. Van Praag, H.M. The significance of dopamine for the mode of action of neuroleptics and the pathogenesis of schizophrenia. *British Journal of Psychiatry*, 1977, *130*, 463–474.
20. Gruen, P.H., Sachar, E.J., Langer, G., Altman, N., Leifer, M., Frantz, A., & Halpern, F.S. Prolactin-responses to neuroleptics in normal and schizophrenic subjects. *Archives General Psychiatry*, 1978, *35*, 108–116.
21. Crow, T.J. Molecular pathology of schizophrenia: more than one disease process? *British Medical Journal*, 1980, *280*, 66–68.
22. Johnstone, E., Crow, T.J., Frith, C.D., Carvey, M.W.P., & Price, J.C. Antipsychotic effect in the treatment of acute schizophrenia. *Lancet*, 1976, *i*, 848–851.
23. Fink, M. Is ECT a useful therapy in schizophrenia? In J.P. Brady & H.K.H. Brodie (Eds.) *Controversy in Psychiatry*. Philadelphia; W.B. Saunders, 1978.
24. Creese, I., Burt, D.R. & Snyder, S.A. Dopamine receptor binding predicts clinical and pharmacological potencies of antischizophrenic drugs. *Science*, 1976, *192*, 481–483.

Part IV

PSYCHOSOCIAL FACTORS AND MENTAL HEALTH SERVICES

Chapter 14

THE MENTAL HEALTH CARE SYSTEM IN TRANSITION

A Study in Organization, Effectiveness, and Costs of Complementary Care for Schizophrenic Patients

Heinz Häfner, M.D., Ph.D. and
Wolfram an der Heiden, M.S.

J.K. Wing[1] has recently reviewed 30 years of psychiatric care in the United Kingdom. Referring to his own evaluative studies, he stated that a large proportion of the long-term hospital stays practiced until the 1950s were unnecessary. Meanwhile a large number of long-stay patients have been rehabilitated and the average duration of stay in mental hospitals has decreased remarkably. In fact, during the last 30 years, the rate of occupied beds has decreased by roughly one-half in England and Wales— from about 3.5 to about 1.8 percent.

An analogous trend can be observed in many countries which have a comparatively large number of long-stay hospital patients and sufficient resources for establishing a complementary mental health care system. Where this has not been the case, for example in Japan, the development seems to have taken an

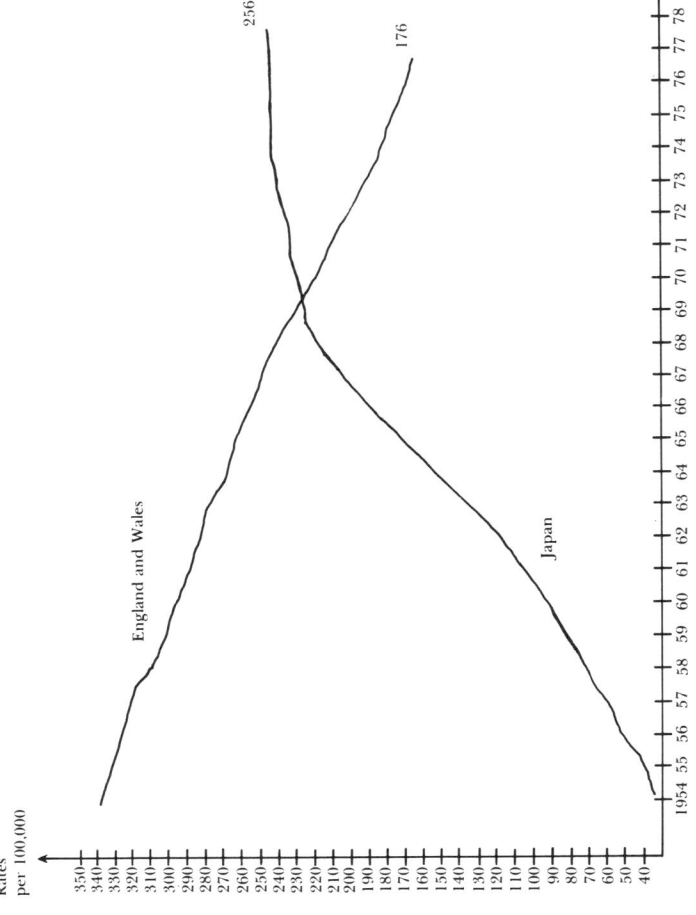

Figure 14-1.   Resident patients in mental illness hospitals and units: England and Wales 31 December 1954–1978 (public + private hospitals).[28]

England and Wales 1954–1977[29] / Japan from 1954–1978 (public + private hospitals).[28]

opposite course, similar to what happened in Europe before 1950 (see Fig. 14-1).

In community mental health services with a sufficient capacity of complementary facilities monitored on the basis of case registers, the rate of occupied psychiatric beds now stands at 1 to 2 per 1000 population aged fifteen to sixty-five.[2-4] Moreover, the recently published statistics from eight case register areas in Great Britain 1976–1981 show an astonishingly uniform trend in the annual rates of treated prevalence.[5] In four of the five registers disposing of figures covering the entire period of observation, treated prevalence amounted to 1.5 to 1.6 percent of the population, whereas in the fifth, Oxford, it was slightly lower at 1.3 percent. The uniformity of the British health care system may largely account for the similarity of the rates.*

The changes in mental health care in the last 30 years have mainly been due to the fundamental reorientation in the care of chronic schizophrenics. In the 1950s in many countries, such as the U.S.A. over 50 percent of the psychiatric beds were still occupied by schizophrenic patients, and 60 to 80 percent of the patients hospitalized for over 1 year belonged to this diagnostic group. Their fate as long-term patients directed attention to the adverse effects of custodial care. To offer better and more humane care for chronic schizophrenics was one of the main objectives in developing complementary services in the community. The favorable results achieved through neuroleptic medication in the treatment of the psychotic symptomatology and the abnormal behavior of schizophrenic patients have made the transition from closed hospital based care possible for the majority of chronic schizophrenics. Another motive for the change to open extramural care stems from the current ideological trend

---

*Distributed over age decades, only the rates for treated prevalence in higher age groups differ more markedly in the register areas. Differences in the mental health care system, for instance regarding the number of places provided by nursing homes for the elderly and the proportion of patients with dementia cared for in homes, exert an essential influence on the utilization of a mental health service.[6]

in public opinion, above all in the Western countries, which demands unlimited autonomy for all and consequently also for psychiatric patients. This, however, in spite of being very helpful in the reform of mental health care in general, often results in less protection and security for the patients and has also consequences for the organization of mental health services, which will be dealt with later.

In many countries the facilities providing complementary care, such as sheltered homes or workshops, are not part of the health care system, nor are they run by psychiatrists. The crucial question whether the objectives, provided adequate extramural care in quantitative and qualitative terms is available, are genuinely attainable or only at the cost of increased deterioration and more frequent relapses, has not yet been answered satisfactorily.

We have made an attempt to answer these questions and to compare step by step the costs of complementary care with those of intramural care provided for schizophrenics. The study was based on the Mannheim community mental health service.

Figure 14-2 illustrates the present topographic situation: A day-hospital, sheltered homes, group homes, apartments, and sheltered workshops have been located in different parts of the city, mainly in good residential areas, in order to prevent the mentally ill from being subjected to segregation and stigmatization anew. However, we have to be aware—as shown by some experience in the U.S.A. and also in the FRG—that complementary facilities for chronic mental patients can be neglected and stigmatized in the same way as was the old mental hospital in the past. The Department for Community Psychiatry at the CIMH has helped to plan and set up all the complementary services now available in Mannheim; it advises them and coordinates the care provided for the patients.

Figure 14-3 illustrates the development of complementary places of care in the period 1976–1984.

At present there are 213 complementary places for adult psychiatric patients, of which 153 are in 5 psychiatric homes and 60 in 7 sheltered group homes or apartments; as well as 120 places in 2 sheltered workshops available in the city with a total population of 305,000. The need for sheltered accommoda-

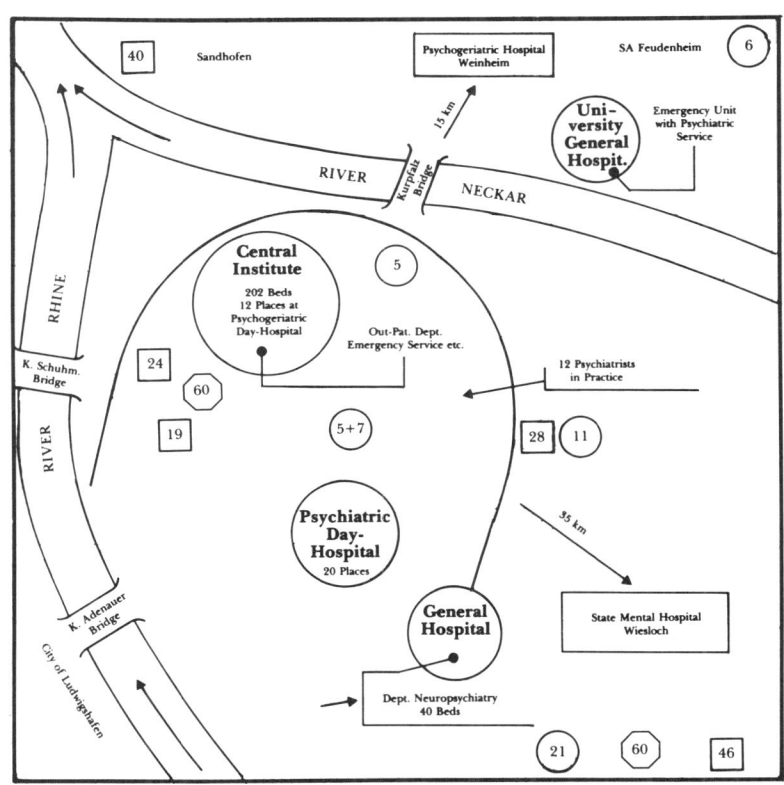

Total number of places

Sheltered homes:	153	Sheltered apartments:	55	Sheltered workshops:	120
Home in Sandhofen	40	Freudenheim	6	F7 (centre)	60
Käthe Luther-Home	19	K4 (centre)	5	Am Sandrain	60
Elisab. Lutz-Home	24	Q4 (centre)	5+7		
St. Anna-Home	46	In association with			
Arbeiterwohlfahrt		the Elisab. Lutz-Home	11		
(a social security		Am Sandrain	21		
organization)	24				

**Figure 14-2.   Mental health facilities serving
Mannheim; City of Mannheim**

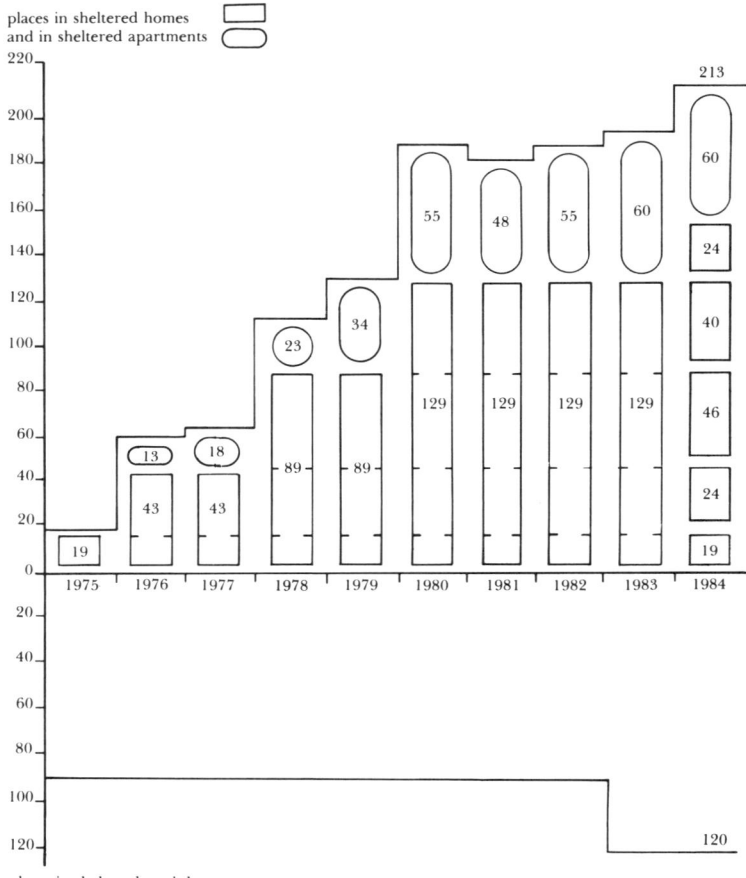

places in sheltered homes
and in sheltered apartments

places in sheltered workshops

**Figure 14-3.   Implementation of complementary
facilities for chronic psychiatric patients
in Mannheim 1975–1984.**

tion, such as homes, seems to have been met for the time being, whereas the need for places in sheltered workshops still exceeds the supply by almost 100 percent.

Inpatient care for adult patients is provided jointly by the Psychiatric Department of the CIMH, which is situated in the city center and which has 106 beds and 32 day-hospital places, and a mental state hospital, some 30 km away from the city center, with 1280 beds (of which about 200 are reserved for patients from Mannheim).

At the current stage in the development of complementary services, only approximately 40 percent of the long-term schizophrenic patients are cared for in psychiatric hospital (1980), as our case register data show. Only one-quarter of the schizophrenic patients requiring treatment for 1 year and more commence such a stay in a psychiatric hospital, whereas three-quarters are admitted for a stay of 1 year or more in complementary services (see Figure 14-4).

DIFFERENCES IN THE ORGANIZATION OF INTRA- AND EXTRAMURAL CARE

Chronic schizophrenics as a rule suffer from deficiencies and disabilities that affect their job performance and social behavior. Depending on the severity and profile of their disability, they need therapeutic measures and/or support at five different levels (see Figure 14-5).

For a long time, the mental hospital alone used to provide more or less adequate care for the chronic patients at all five levels. This is why Goffman[7] has termed it a total institution. In a complementary service system the functions are separated.

Medication and psychotherapy are, in general, administered by a psychiatric outpatient department or by private psychiatrists. Accommodation is provided by halfway houses or residential homes; work and occupation by sheltered workshops; while patients' clubs, lay initiatives, etc., are responsible for the furtherance of social contacts and leisure activities.

The fact differing needs for care are met by different facilities, some operating independently of each other and financed from different sources, has consequences. The patients, in particular the severely disordered, utilize a whole network of services. In ideal circumstances their individual needs are met; at worst, the measures are badly organized and the objectives of therapy inconsistent. The reality in patient care surely lies somewhere between these poles.

Where mental health care crosses the boundary of social

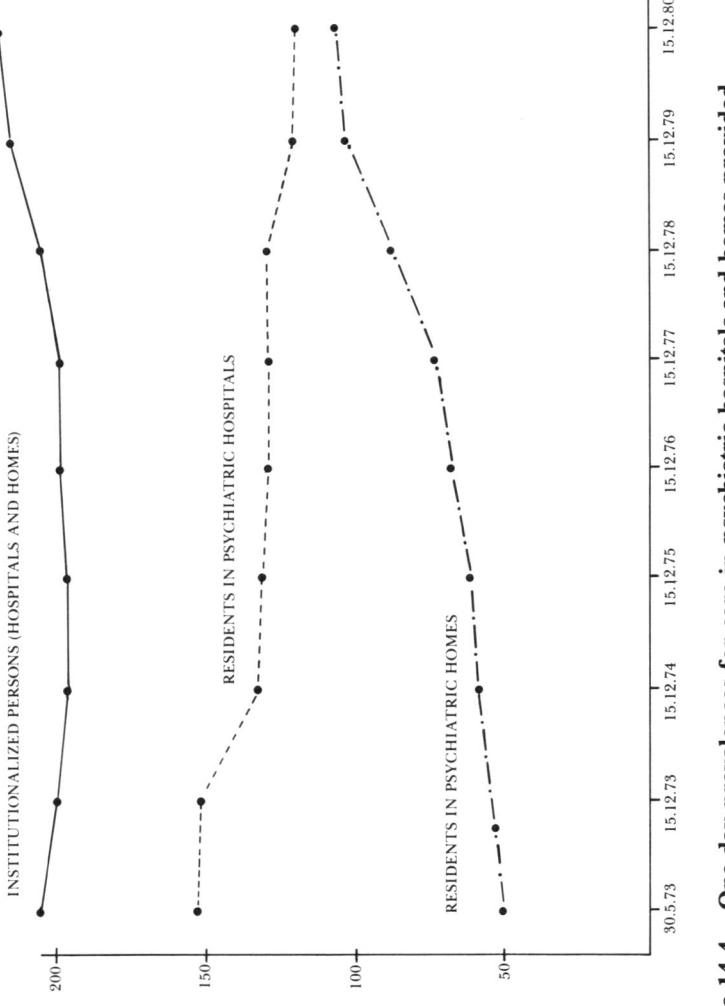

Figure 14-4. One-day prevalences for care in psychiatric hospitals and homes provided for patients with schizophrenia (I.C.D. No. 295) 1973–1980.

**Figure 14-5. Levels of Need for Care
of the Chronically Mentally Ill and Disabled.**

*Long-Term
Hospital Care*

Level of Need

Community Care

Care Offered By:

Psychiatric Treatment	Psychiatric Outpatient Care
Accommodation	Home, Sheltered Apartment, etc.
Work, Occupation	Sheltered Workshop, etc.
Social Contacts	Patient Club
Leisure-Time Activity	Lay Initiative

Care
Offered
By:

Mental Hospital

care for basic human needs, as in some poverty programs in the USA in the early 1950s and at Trieste at present, the situation may be very different in this respect. We have investigated the functioning and efficiency of the services in Mannheim at two levels:

1.   At a global level by using case register data, but limiting our study to the utilization of mental health services. At this level changes in the overall service system and in the utilization of individual services were recorded and rough indicators for the distribution of case load, and for the effectiveness and the costs of the measures were worked out.
2.   At a more detailed level, confined to certain homogeneous patient groups with definable needs for care and comparable dimensions of psychopathology, by means of representative cohort studies. They enabled us to record all utilizations per case, i.e. not only those of psychiatric services, but also of general practitioners and social services, and to calculate the direct costs and to assess the effectiveness of the service delivery.[8-12]

QUANTITATIVE DESCRIPTION OF THE COMPLEX PATTERN OF CARE FOR CHRONIC SCHIZOPHRENICS

In order to quantify the complex patterns of care, an der Heiden and Klug[13] at our Institute have developed a method enabling us to record all utilizations per case of all services in a given period of time with the help of the so-called utilization raster. By using the two-dimensional matrix based on 14-day intervals, it is possible to describe the entire pattern of course of service utilizations.

Taking all the Mannheim inhabitants who had been admitted to a psychiatric hospital with the diagnosis of schizophrenia (ICD295) in a 1-year period as our basis, we followed a cohort of 148 patients over 1 1/2 years. Table 14-1 depicts the average utilization of the various service categories available to all patients in the follow-up period in comparable rates (nursing days

Table 14-1. Rates of Intra- and Extramural Care

Institution	N (Patients)	Average Rate per 100 Patients and Year*
Psychiatric Hospital	148	9270 Days
Day-/Night-Hospital	6	284 Days
Sheltered Homes	38	4700 Days
Sheltered Workshops	36	2560 Days
Psychiatric Out-Patient Department		485 Contacts
Psychiatrists in Free Practice	136	915 Contacts
Other Physicians		460 Contacts
Patients' Clubs and Miscellaneous	67	245 Contacts

* The calculation of the rates is based on a total of 148 patients.
Source: Hafner, H. + an der Heiden, W. The impact of changing systems of care on patterns of utilization by schizophrenics. *Social Psychiatry*, 1983, *18*, 153–160.

per 100 patients per year or outpatient contacts per 100 patients per year).

In accordance with the multifarious needs of the mentally ill and disabled, multiple utilizations (i.e. one patient utilizing more than one service) predominate. However, it was not possible to identify "typical" combinations. Among the total of 3,858 14-day intervals spent outside the mental hospital the following patterns turned out to be the most frequent:

1. residential home in combination with outpatient psychiatric care and

2. sheltered workshop in combination with outpatient psychiatric care,

both patterns accounting for only 11 percent and 10 percent of the total of intervals respectively.

STUDIES ON THE EFFECTIVENESS OF COMPLEMENTARY CARE

Does a varying intensity of complementary care influence the risk of relapse?

The objectives of complementary care are defined as the avoidance of unnecessary hospitalizations and the shortening of the inevitable ones.[cf. 14] The degree of goal attainment can be measured by the shortening of hospital stays, the reduction of readmission rates, and the extension of the time spent outside mental hospital.[15] Although these outcome criteria are problematic in isolated consideration,[16] they provide important information about the functioning of a complementary service system. If other independent variables, such as living conditions and length of illness, and outcome criteria at the patient level, such as the psychiatric symptomatology and behavior, are taken into account simultaneously, the evaluation of complementary care provides information on the success or failure of such a system and on the outcome of the patients.

Owing to the complexity and heterogeneity of the patterns of care utilized by our sample, it was not possible to compare "typical" patient careers in complementary services with regard to effectiveness. To start with general indicators of intervention and its efficacy, we first studied the influence of the intensity of extramural care upon the probability of readmission (see Figure 14-6). For this purpose we divided the 80 cohort patients who had been readmitted at least once in the follow-up period of 18 months into three equal groups according to the number of contacts with complementary services after discharge. For each group we then calculated the probability of readmission within 1 year after discharge.

For group 3, showing the most intensive utilization, the cu-

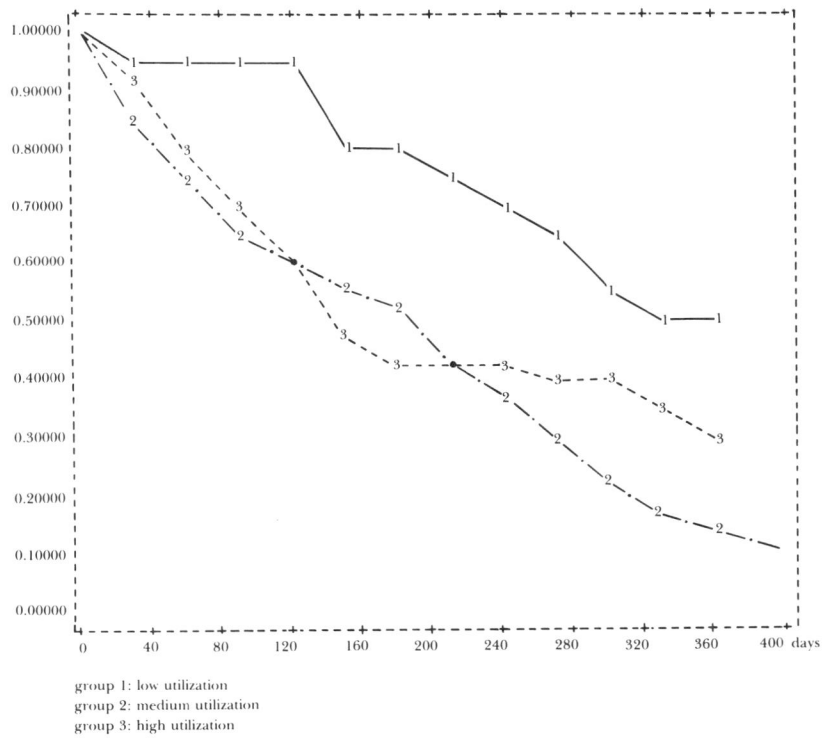

group 1: low utilization
group 2: medium utilization
group 3: high utilization

**Figure 14-6.   The influence of extramural care on the
probability of readmission.**

mulative probability of not being rehospitalized after 1 year was
p= .30; for group 2, characterized by a medium intensity of utilization, it was as low as p= .14. Group 1 was not comparable,
because it comprised patients with illnesses of short length and
favorable prognosis. This means that in the group of predominantly chronic schizophrenia an intensive utilization of complementary mental health services is associated with a slightly
lower probability of readmission (at least for 1 year).

THE EFFECTIVENESS OF SELECTED COMPONENTS OF THE CARE PROVIDED
FOR SCHIZOPRHENICS

Considering the complexity of complementary care, the question arises which of the components—for instance, accommodation in a residential home, or psychiatric outpatient therapy—actually influence the course of the illness and possibly also the social course, and which merely increase or reduce comfort in the life of the ill. To answer these questions there are, however, as yet only few results available.

As shown by Table 14-1, outpatient medical care plays an important role in community care: Out of 148 patients, 136 had, at differing frequencies, contacted the psychiatric outpatient department or private psychiatrists when not hospitalized. A further analysis of our data* focused precisely on this component of complementary care. To answer the question, "How does outpatient care influence (1) the course of the illness— measured by the psychiatric symptomatology, and (2) the frequency and length of readmission?" we collected data on utilization, demography, former inpatient care, and the mental status of the patients. A PSE interview[17] was administered at four points during the follow-up period. Given these additional variables, we were able to control for the duration of illness prior to the patients' entry into our study,[18] for family and social environment[19–24] and for mental status as well as for the effect of the service variables on the outcome of complementary care. In order to identify the direction of this relation, we correlated the data obtained in the first 12 months with the corresponding data collected between the thirteenth and eighteenth month. The influence of the intervening variables mentioned was excluded by partial correlation. (Figure 14-7). Our results show that an intensification—number of contacts per time interval— and an increased proportion of outpatient care in total psychiatric care reduce the total length of hospital readmissions. This

---

*Including all contacts of the cohort patients with the psychiatric outpatient service of the CIMH, private psychiatrists, or some other physician, if the treatment received was due to the mental illness (cf. Table 14-l).

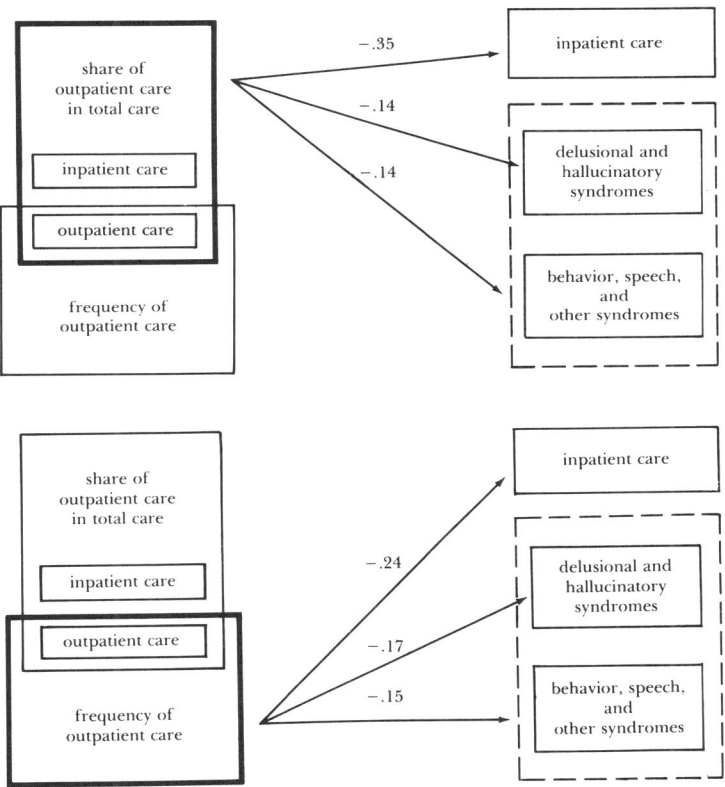

Figure 14-7. Impact of psychiatric outpatient care on readmissions and on symptomatology in schizophrenia—psychopathology, length of treatment, and living conditions considered.

means that more psychiatric outpatient care for chronic schizophrenic patients, in fact, reduces, instead of increasing, the need for hospital treatment. Moreover, the intensification of outpatient psychiatric treatment reduces the probability of productive symptoms (PSE subscore DAH) as well as behavioral and speech disorders (PSE subscore BSO) in schizophrenic patients. To interpret these results we assume that the higher compliance of the patients consulting medical services more often and, as a consequence of it, the higher continuity in neuroleptic medication are important factors influencing the variable "intensity of extramural care." Since both the degree of the symptomatology and the total length of inpatient treatment prior to the follow-up period were controlled for, it can be ruled out that the results are confounded by the variable "severity of illness."

COST ANALYSIS OF THE COMMUNITY CARE FOR SCHIZOPHRENICS

Besides the effectiveness, the costs of a system of complementary care, compared with those of the traditional one, are of interest. We have, therefore, compared the direct costs of community care with those of a permanent stay in a mental hospital over an equal period of time on the basis of the utilization data derived from our patient cohort.[25, 26] Contrary to the practice in comprehensive cost-effectiveness analysis, we have confined ourselves to calculating the direct costs for two reasons:

First, the economic questions we are interested in are limited: namely, what are the costs accruing from typical complementary care as compared with permanent hospital stays in the case of chronic schizophrenics? Such a comparison is more informative if the calculation is based only on the total current expenses of each service form, which are definable according to the contemporary psychiatric consensus. The calculation loses its informative value for our purpose inasmuch as capital expenditure or indirect costs, differing markedly in national or local terms, such as depreciation of buildings or pension payments, are included.

Secondly, if the highly varying capital expenditure and indirect costs were included, the small size of the sample would lead to considerable distortions and consequently to results no longer useful to us.

The total costs per patient are made up of the direct costs resulting from hospital, day-hospital, and night-hospital care; from the accommodation and care provided in psychiatric homes or sheltered group homes; from the utilization of sheltered workshops and rehabilitation facilities as well as from medical treatment (covered by the social insurance scheme). The arithmetic mean of the total costs of extramural care amount to 15,574 DM over 1 year (see Figure 14-8). A 1-year uninterrupted stay in the local mental hospital cost 36,497 DM. Thus, the costs of the community care for schizophrenics over one year averaged only 43 percent of the costs of a 1-year stay in the mental hospital. And of the total costs of the community care provided for schizophrenics, almost 80 percent resulted from hospitalizations due to relapses. This statement of a higher economic efficiency of extramural care, which possesses validity at least with respect to its tendency, but which is still marred by inexactitudes, is further supported by the fact that out of a total of 145 patients who were temporarily discharged from the mental hospital and who received extramural care during the follow-up period, only in the case of 7 patients were the costs higher than if these patients had been cared for in mental hospital.

When concluding that extramural care of schizophrenics is altogether more effective, it has to be borne in mind that this applies only provided quantitatively, and qualitatively adequate services are available. When further concluding that extramural care is also more economical than long-term hospital treatment, the conclusion, strictly speaking, applies only to the cost structure of the Federal Republic of Germany. It is not applicable to mental health care systems characterized by different systems of funding.

CONSEQUENCES FOR THE ORGANIZATION OF COMPLEMENTARY CARE

Finally, I would like to come back to an essential aspect of the quality of extramural care. The organization of the various treatment and rehabilitation services as several independent facilities, mentioned at the outset, necessitates coordination of the measures on the individual patient and cooperation for guaranteeing appropriate care for all patients. The fulfillment of this important task, however, if hindered by the zeitgeist demanding unlimited autonomy—and in the Netherlands, by tradition. Such thinking is particularly deeply rooted in the field of com-

partial hospitalization———————— 191.—(1.2%)

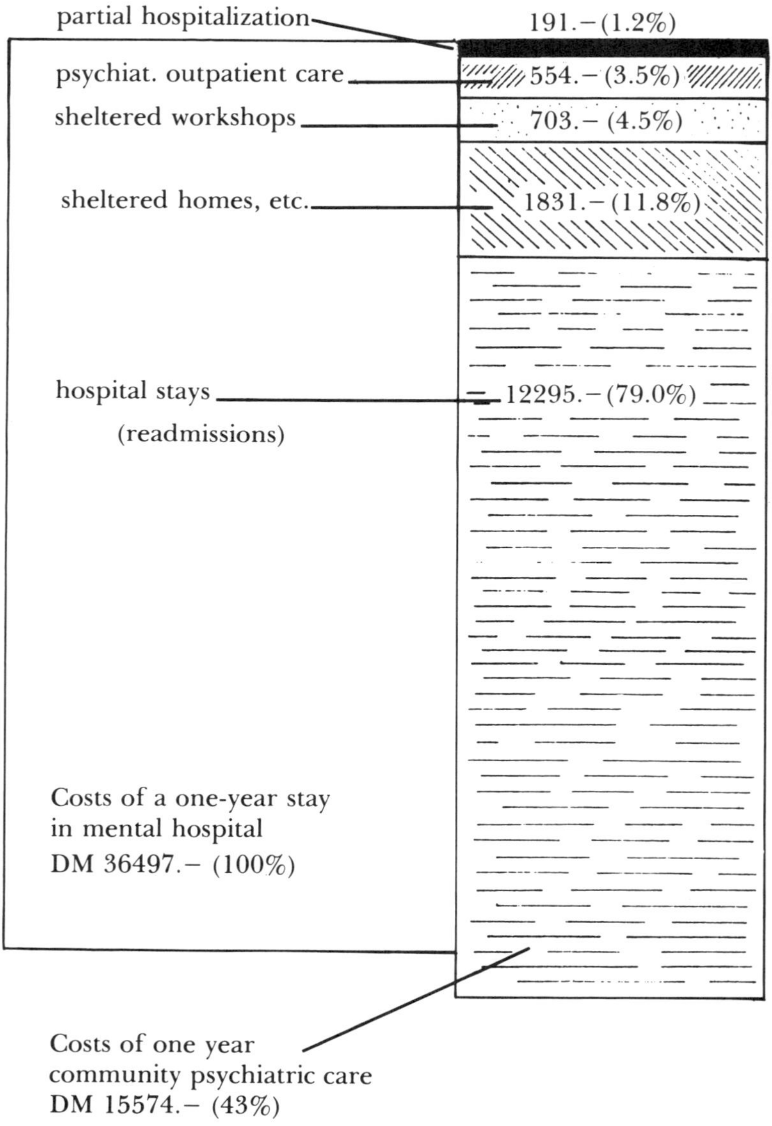

psychiat. outpatient care _____ 554.— (3.5%)

sheltered workshops _____ 703.— (4.5%)

sheltered homes, etc. _____ 1831.— (11.8%)

hospital stays _____ 12295.— (79.0%)

(readmissions)

Costs of a one-year stay
in mental hospital
DM 36497.— (100%)

Costs of one year
community psychiatric care
DM 15574.— (43%)

**Figure 14-8. Costs of a one-year stay in mental hospital
compared with one year total costs of
community mental health care.**

munity mental health care. The goal of providing uniform patterns of rehabilitation and treatment for the mentally ill within the comunity health care system can only be reached if the agencies or persons in question relinquish their claim for unlimited autonomy.

Regardless of the fact that a large proportion of chronic patients is leaving the mental health care system, it still remains the task of psychiatric research to develop better methods of primary and secondary prevention, in order to facilitate the life of these patients and to prevent the development or chronification of disabling illnesses like schizophrenia. For this purpose it is necessary to cross the boundary of the academic setting and to overcome the limits set to the responsibility of the health care system, which, however, has so far proved extremely difficult for psychiatric research, other than in Greece.

In the last 2 decades, psychiatry has made decisive progress in the fields of diagnosis, therapy, and epidemiological research. Now this progress has to be translated into improved service programs, facilities, and systems. At the same time, high standard service research needs to be increased, in order to provide empirically better founded and more rational basis for the planning and organization of a changing service system and to guard the patients against unrealistic ideologies and, on the other hand, also against professional egotism.

REFERENCES

1. Wing, J. K. Mental health services in the United Kingdom. Paper presented at the Symposium on Mental Health Service Research, VII World Congress of Psychiatry, Vienna, 13 July, 1983.
2. Fryers, T. Psychiatric in-patients in 1982—how many beds? *Psychological Medicine*, 1974, *4*, 196–211.
3. Häfner, H. & Klug, J. The impact of an expanding community mental health service on patterns of bed usage: Evaluation of four-year period of implementation. *Psychological Medicine*, 1982, *12* 177–190.
4. Dupont, A. & Weeke, A. Antallet af psykiatriske indlæggelser i Danmark. *Ugeskrift for Läger*, 1977, *139*, 1241–1242.

5. Gibbons, J. L., Jennings, E. & Wing, J. K. Psychiatric care in 8 register areas. Statistics from eight psychiatric case registers in Great Britain 1976–1981. Southamptom; The University of Southampton, 1983.

6. Strömgren, E., Kyst, E., Ryberg, I., et al: Estimation of need on the basis of field survey findings. In *Estimating needs for mental health care: A contribution of epidemiology*. (Ed.) H. Hafner Berlin, Springer, 1979.

7. Goffman, E. *Asylums: Essays on the social situation of mental patients and other inmates*. Garden City: Anchor, Doubleday, 1961.

8. Häfner, H., & Klug, J. First evaluation of the Mannheim community mental health service. In Epidemiological research as basis for the organization of extramural psychiatry. E. Strömgren (Ed.) *Acta Psychiatrica Scandinavica*, 1980, Supplement 285 (Vol. 62) 68–78.

9. Häfner, H., & Klug, J. Wissenschaftliche Begleitung der Entwicklung einer gemeindenahen psychiatrischen Versorgung in Mannheim. In H. J. Haase, (Ed.) *Bürgernahe Psychiatrie im Wirkungsbereich des psychiatrischen Krankenhauses*. Erlangen, perimed Fachbuch-Verlagsgessellschaft, 1981.

10. Häfner, H. & an der Heiden, W. Evaluation gemeindenaher Versorgung psychisch Kranker. Ergebnisse von 4 Jahren wissenschaftlicher Begleitung der Aufbauphase des Mannheimer Modells. *Archiv für Psychiatrie und Nervenkrankheiten*, 1982, *232*, 71–95.

11. Häfner, H. & an der Heiden, W. The impact of a changing system of care on patterns of utilization by schizophrenics. *Social Psychiatry*, 1983, *18*, 153–160.

12. an der Heiden, W. & Krumm, B. Does outpatient treatment reduce hospital stay in schizophrenics? *European Archives of Psychiatry and Neurological Sciences*. (In press).

13. an der Heiden, W. & Klug, J. An integrated record system for the observation of the demand for medical and social aftercare as basis for organizing extramural services. *Acta Psychiatrica Scandinavica*, 1980, *62*, Supplement *285* 54–59.

14. Bericht über die Lage der Psychiatrie in der Bundesrepublik Deutschland - Zur psychiatrischen und psychotherapeutisch/psychosomatischen Versorgung der Bevölkerung. Deutscher Bundestag, Drs. 7/4200, 7/4201, Bonn, 1975.

15. Erickson, R. G. Outcome studies in mental hospitals: A review. *Psychological Bulletin*, 1975, *82*, 519–540.

16. Kunze, H. *Psychiatrische Übergangseinrichtungen und Heime*. Stuttgart; Enke Verlag, 1981.

17. Wing, J. K., Cooper, J. E. & Sartorius, N. *Measurement and classification of psychiatric symptoms: An instruction manual for PSE and Catago Program*. London; Cambridge University Press, 1974.

18. Rosenblatt, A., & Mayer, J. The recidivism of mental patients: A review of past studies. *American Journal of Orthopsychiatry*, 1974, *44*, 697–706.

19. Brown, G. W., Carstairs, G. M. & Topping, G. C. The post-hospital adjustment of chronic mental patients. *Lancet*, 1958, 685–689.

20. Brown, G. W., Monck, E. M., Carstairs, G. M. et al: The influence of family life on the course of schizophrenic illness. *British Journal of Prevention and Social Medicine*, 1962, *16*, 58–68.

21. Brown, G. W., Birley, J. L. T., & Wing, J. K. The influence of family life on the course of schizophrenic disorders: A replication. *British Journal of Psychiatry*, 1972, *12*, 241–258.

22. Vaughn, C. E. & Leff, J. The measurement of expressed emotion in the families of psychiatric patients. *British Journal of Social and Clinical Psychiatry*, 1976, *15*, 157–165.

23. Vaughn, C. E., & Leff, J. The influence of family and social factors on the course of psychiatric illness: A comparison of schizophrenic and depressed neurotic patients. *British Journal of Psychiatry*, 1976, *129*, 125–137.

24. Blumenthal, R., Kreisman, D. & O'Connor, P. A. Return to the family and its consequence for rehospitalization among recently discharged mental patients. *Psychological Medicine*, 1982, *12*, 141–147.

25. Bardens, R. Kostenanalyse bei Nachsorgeeinrichtungen für schizophrene Patieten. Unpublished doctoral dissertation, University of Mannheim, 1984.

26. Häfner, H. an der Heiden, W., Buchholz, W. et al. Organisation, Wirksamkeit und Wirtschaftlichkeit komplementärer Versorgung Schizophrener. *Nervenarzt* In press.

27. Häfner, H. & an der Heiden, W. Evaluation of long-term community care for patients with schizophrenia. In T. Helgason *The*

long-term treatment of functional psychoses. Cambridge; University Press, 1984.

28. Takahashi, S. Personal communication, 1980.
29. Department of Health and Social Security. Inpatient statistics from the Mental Health Enquiry for England. Statistical and Research Reports Series No. 26, 1980. H.M.S.O., London.

Chapter 15

DECENTRALIZATION, SECTORIZATION AND THE DEVELOPMENT OF ALTERNATIVES TO INSTITUTIONAL CARE IN A NORTHERN COUNTY IN SWEDEN

Carlo Perris, M.D.

There is hardly any other sector of the health care system that is going through such a radical change in its organization as that concerning mental health.

If the nineteenth century can be regarded as the period when the mental health movement started to reach its peak at the turn of the century, the second half of the twentieth century will be remembered as the epoch when an opposite trend became dominant. In fact, traditional mental hospitals are being successively dismantled in most industrialized countries and their use for the treatment of the mentally ill is regarded as more damaging than as effective.

A key concept behind the transformation of the organization of psychiatric care that is under way is that of "deinstitutionalization." It has been defined by Brown[1] as follows:

1. Release to the community of all institutional patients who have been given adequate preparation for such a change;
2. Prevention of inappropriate mental hospital admis-

sions through the provision of community alternatives for treatment;

3. Establishment and maintenance of community support systems for noninstitutionalized persons receiving mental health services in the community.

It should be noted that this definition is much broader than that used in everyday language and that refers mainly to the discharge of long-stay patients from the mental hospitals. Brown's definition, in fact, takes into account, not only the release of institutionalized patients, but also the prevention of new admissions, and the need of creating supportive agencies in the community for those people in need of psychiatric assistance. An even more comprehensive interpretation of the concept of deinstitutionalization, akin to some of the ideological tenets behind the Italian psychiatric reform[2] encompasses efforts aimed at avoiding the fact that various kinds of deviant behavior are unwarrantedly comprised within the domain of psychiatry, understood here as one of the "institutions" for social control.

Unfortunately, the common understanding of the term deinstitutionalization mentioned above is not without foundation. In fact, it seems that the release of long-stay patients from the mental hospitals represents the most conspicous expression of the changing orientation in psychiatric care, whereas both the "adequate preparation" of the patients to be released, and the development of alternatives to institutional care advocated by Brown have been neglected to a very large extent. Bachrach,[3] in commenting on the definition of deinstitutionalization given by Brown, did not hesitate to regard it as "ideal." A very common pattern has been that unprepared long-stay patients have been released to the community long before any adequate alternative system of care had been developed.

Although there are common values in the planning and implementing of deinstitutionalization, there are, obviously, also differences among different countries either as concerns the pace with which such process is carried out, or as concerns the attention paid to development of alternative structures for the care of the mentally ill.

Sweden is one of the countries where the dismantling of traditional hospitals is going on at a slower pace than in other countries, and where the development of alternative structures is expected to occur prior to the release of hospitalized patients. Also, much concern is shown for the preparation of patients expected to be deinstitutionalized.

A however, cursory survey of the process of change in the organization of psychiatric care in Sweden would be beyond the scope of this chapter. Thus, I will exemplify this process by reporting the organizational changes that have occurred in one of the Swedish counties where I have a first hand experience.

THE COUNTY OF VÄSTERBOTTEN: ITS MAIN CHARACTERISTICS AND THE STATE OF MENTAL CARE BEFORE THE PROCESS OF REFORM

The County of Västerbotten (Figure 15-1) is the second most northern county in Sweden. It covers an area of about 55,000 square kilometers and has a population short of 245,000 inhabitants. There are three main towns, Umeå, Skellefteå, and Lycksele, where most of the population is concentrated. The county is divided into three main health districts with a general hospital in each of the above mentioned towns. The general hospital at Umeå is also a teaching hospital and has, for some of the specialities, a regional responsibility covering a population of about 1 million people. There is a fair network of primary care units, but the distance from the main centers to the most remote villages amounts to hundreds of kilometers.

Details about the organization of psychiatric care prior to the process of reform have been given elsewhere;[4-6] thus only the main characteristics will be summarized here. Traditionally, all psychiatric care has been concentrated at Umeå where a state mental hospital had been built in 1933, and a small psychiatric department had been active at the general hospital (which became a University Department in 1960). At the periphery, occasional consultations were held at Lycksele and Skellefteå by a travelling psychiatrist within the frame of the community psychiatric unit (*Hjälpverksamheten*) proper of each state hospital.[7]

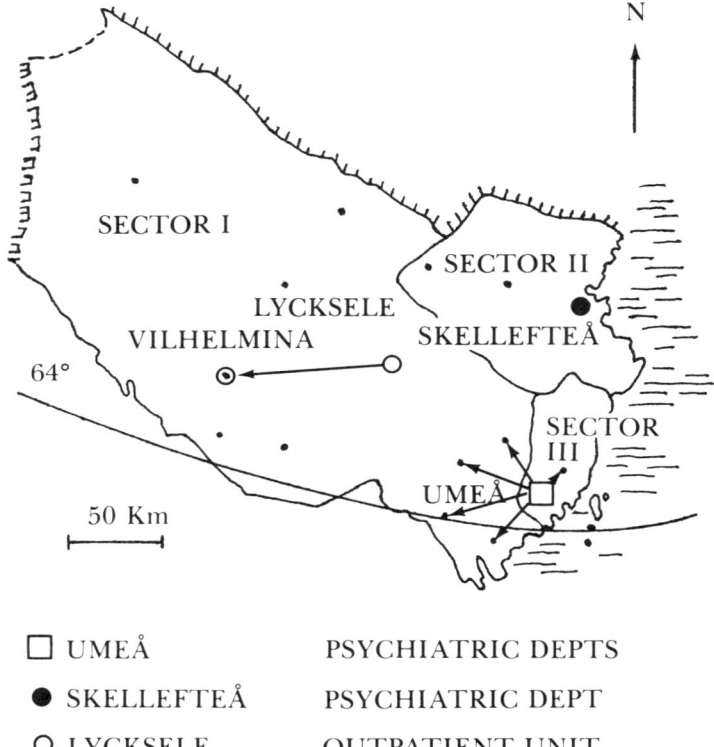

☐ UMEÅ   PSYCHIATRIC DEPTS

● SKELLEFTEÅ   PSYCHIATRIC DEPT

○ LYCKSELE   OUTPATIENT UNIT

⊙ VILHELMINA   OUTPATIENT UNIT

• District doctor(s)

Figure 15-1. **The county of Västerbotten. The figure
shows the division of the county into
three health districts. The Umeå-
psychiatric sector comprises only one part of the
Umeå health district. The difference between the
health districts and the psychiatric sectors is due
to the uneven distribution of inhabitants in the
health districts.**

The process of Restructuring

The first step towards a process of reorganization was taken in 1967, when the responsibility for psychiatric care was transferred from the state to the county authorities, which already had the responsibility for all medical care in their area. Such transfer of responsibility can be regarded also as a first step towards sectorization at the national level. In fact, prior to this administrative change, the responsibility of state mental hospitals very often stretched—as in the case of Västerbotten—beyond the boundaries of single counties.

In 1967, there were about 1,000 patients at the mental hospital at Umeå and, in addition, few hundred more were cared for in psychiatric nursing homes in the Umeå area, or in family care.

The process of reorganization of the psychiatric services that is still going on was first planned early in the 1970s when the following major goals were settled:

a)   A decentralization of services within the county, including the building of a new department at the general hospital in Skellefteå;

b)   A successive reduction of beds in the psychiatric institutions through a process of planned deinstitutionalization;

c)   The development of outpatient services in the county to facilitate the prevention of inappropriate hospital admissions.

In the progress of the reorganization, other goals besides those defined at the start have been added:

d)   The integration of the services at the mental hospital with those at the university department; and

e)   A division of the county into three main sectors, each of them expected to have, at least provisionally, inpatient facilities both at the mental hospital, and at the general (university) hospital.

Between 1972 and 1984 most of the goals defined above had been reached. After some delay, inpatient services in Skellefteå had begun in 1984. Meanwhile, it has been possible to contain, and also reduce the number of admissions, and drastically to reduce the number of inpatients at the various psychiatric facilities. The stages of restructuring are summarized in Table 15-1, whereas the reduction in the number of inpatients is illustrated in Figures 15-2, 15-3, and 15-4. With the exception of 134 geriatric patients, who have been transferred to the department of geriatrics, and who should be regarded as "transinstitutionalized" rather than deinstitutionalized, the marked decrease of long-stay patients has been obtained by the implementation of appropriate, and individualized training programs.

During the last few years, the pace in the transformation process has considerably increased and plans are now being made to phase out the mental hospital completely by 1990.

Organizational Changes in the Umeå Sector

In order to give a closer view of the process of reorganization of psychiatric services, I will illustrate it at a closer range, focusing on the sector that is under my own responsibility.

The Umeå sector is comprised of the town of Umeå and of a neighboring commune with a total population of about 90,000. The demographic characteristics of the sector are shown in Table 15-2 and the psychiatric facilities at present available are shown in Table 15-3. When the sectorization was implemented, there were about 180 beds at the mental hospital which belonged to the Umeå sector. Their successive decrease is shown in Figure 15-5. An additional 20 beds will be eliminated in 1986 when the rehabilitation ward will be closed down and substituted by two smaller (8 beds each) supervised rehabilitation units in the community. A follow-up of the deninstitutionalized patients was carried out in 1983 to assess their quality of life, and to be sure that the patients did not live under poor conditions. Figure 15-6 illustrates the reduction of the long-stay patients (1 year or longer at hospital) and the accumulation of the new long-stay patients that has occurred since 1978. It should be

**Table 15-1.   The Stages of the Process of
Reorganization of Psychiatric Care
in the County of Västerbotten**

1967	Transfer of the responsibility for psychiatric care from the state to the county authority;
1972	Planning of the reorganization of psychiatric care to 1980;
1975	Implementing of a stable outpatient unit at Lycksele;
1977	Implementing of a stable outpatient unit at Skellefteå;
1978	Integration of the services at the mental hospital and at the university department of psychiatry at the general hospital;
1979	Sectorization of the psychiatric services into three sectors;
1984	Implementing of inpatient services at the general hospital in Skellefteå.

mentioned in this last regard that this accumulation is mostly due to referrals to the hospital by decision of the court, with new provisions at present under planning in the whole country. The release of our long-stay patients has been preceded, as described in detail elsewhere[9, 10] by a repeated individual assessment of the needs of each patient and by individualized training programs. The training was started when the patients were still in their original ward and was continued after discharge until it was felt that the patients could be left on their own. A small number among them (n=27) has been trained to live in group homes. A small mobile unit, comprised of two mental nurses and one occupational therapist supervises the patients released to the community and takes care of them whenever needed in a close collaboration with staff members from the social welfare units. The earliest group homes were implemented in 1980; the patients living in them have acquired a high degree of autonomy and require a minimal amount of psychiatric supervision.

Integration of Out- and In-patient services

Inspired by the principles of the Italian psychiatric reform, we have recently integrated our out- and inpatient services in the sense that two teams have been created which have the responsibility for the two subsectors into which our catchment area

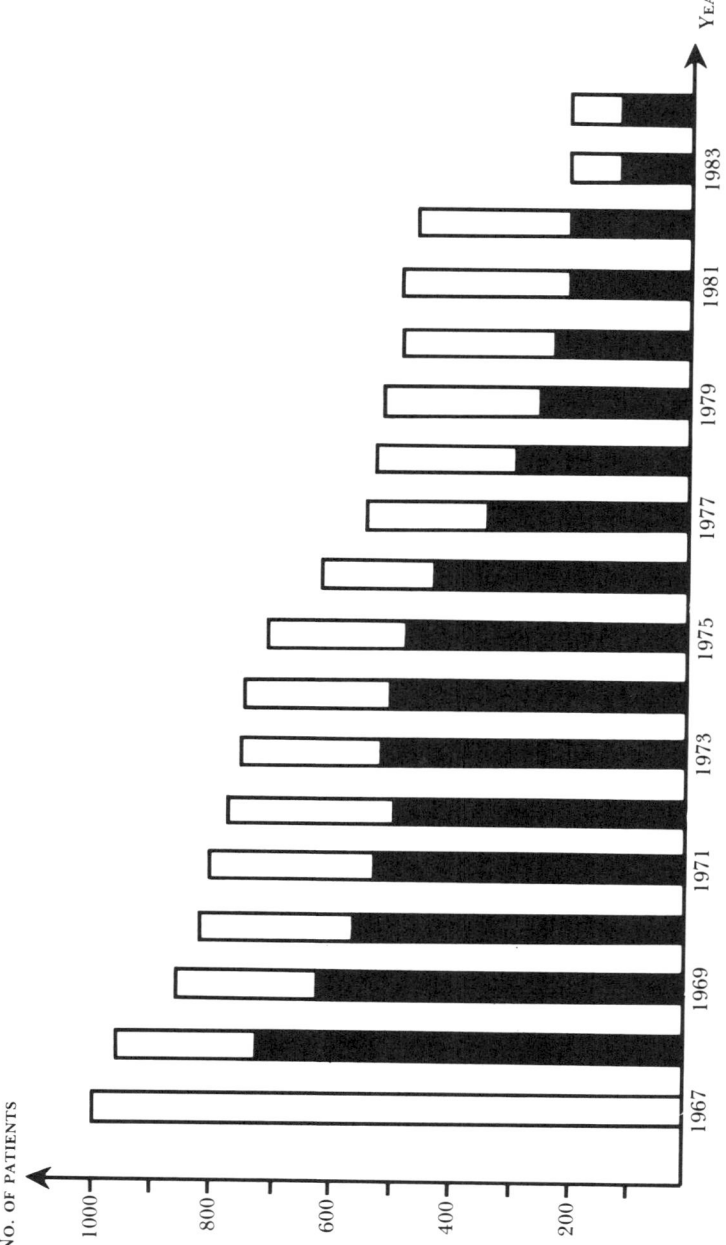

Figure 15-2.   Reduction of the number of inpatients at the mental hospital, 1967–1984.

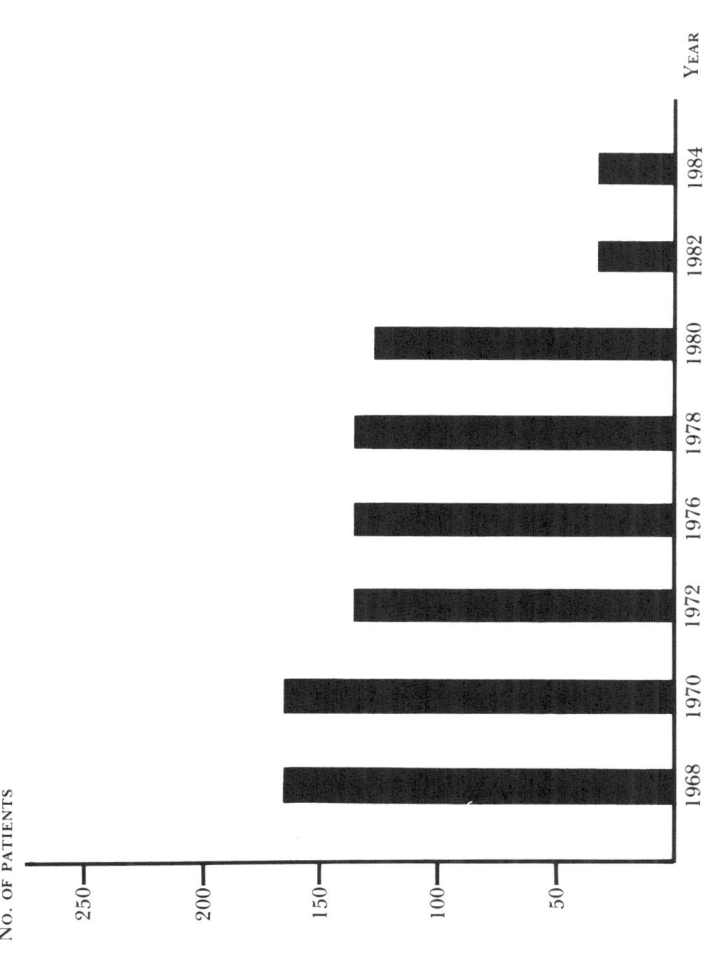

Figure 15-3.   Reduction of the number of psychiatric patients in nursing homes, 1968–1984.

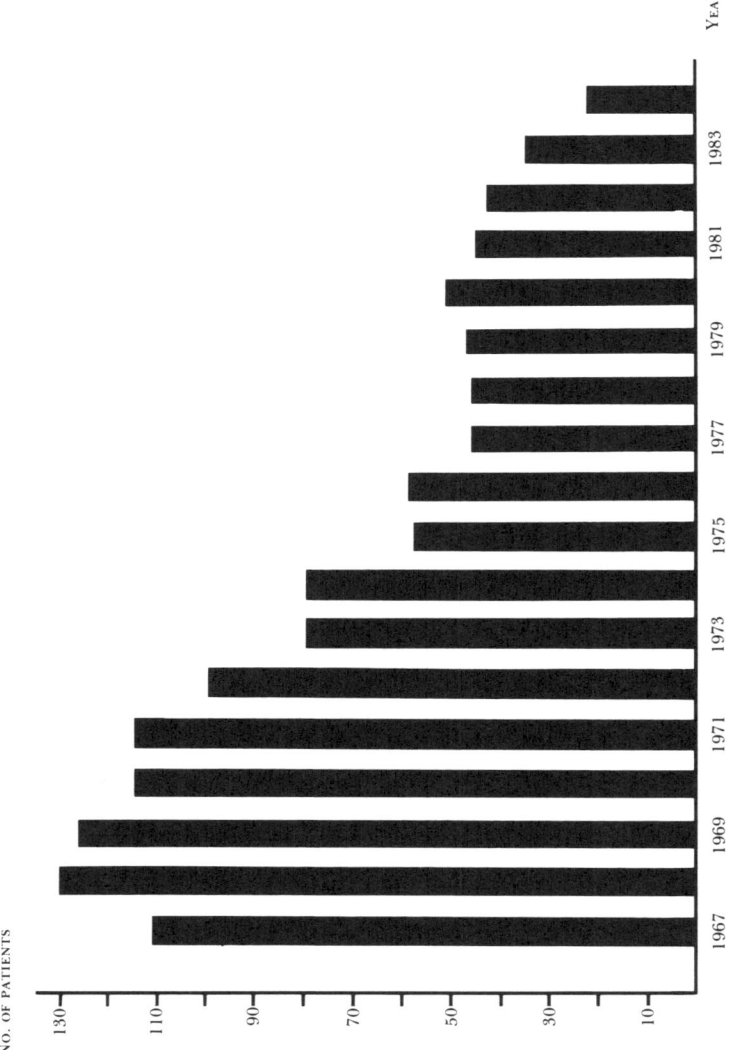

Figure 15-4.   Reduction of the number of patients in family care from 1967–1984.

**Table 15-2.   Demographic Characteristics
of the Umeå Sector**

Population:	86,500 inhabitants (about 70,000 at Umeå)	
Immigrants:	(about) 2,500 (59% Finnish)	
Age distribution (Dec 1983):		
	0–15	18.260
	16–64	56.106
	64–	19.351
Most common type of employment:	Public Services	42%
	Industry	17%
	Commerce	16%

has been divided.[6] Each team serves about 45,000 inhabitants and has a 15-bed acute admission unit at the general hospital as the inpatient resource. All the personnel has been trained for therapeutic tasks so that we can assure each patient an appropriate level of assistance and, what is more important, a far-reaching continuity of care. Since this reform was implemented (in September, 1983), we have been able to reduce the number of admissions by about 11 percent and the length of stay at hospital by about 35 percent (average length = 15 days). Such a shortening of the length of stay has been possible because the same people who have the care of the patients at the ward have also the responsibility of aftercare when the patients are discharged.

CONCLUSIONS

Our experience in a well-defined geographical area suggests that a planned phasing out of a larger mental hospital is feasible and can be achieved within reasonable timelimits.

To avoid negative effects, a careful planning to meet the needs of the released patients has to be made, and the patients have to be trained to be able to cope successfully with the change.

**Table 15-3.   Umeå Sector (90,000 population +
10,000 students and transient residents)**

2 Admission Wards, DGH-Teaching	30 Beds
1 " Geropsychiatry, "	10
1 Rehab. Ward, MH (to be closed 1985)	20
1 Long-Stay Ward, MH (" 1986)	20
1 " Geropsychiatry, MH	20
1 Mixed Security Ward, MH	18
	118 = 1.2/Thousand Population

Other Facilities:

1 Day-Hospital, DGH	About	20 Pat.s
1 Night-Hospital, MH		18 Beds
1 Community-Based Unit (Treatment)		5 "
(1 " " (Rehab.)		6 ")
9 Occasionally Supervised Group Homes		27 Patients
7 Family Care Units		14 "

DGH = District General Hospital (Teaching)
MH = Mental Hospital

The number of beds in acute units can be greatly contained if the personnel at the wards is adequately trained. We believe that a full integration of out- and inpatient services is preferable to a separation of these services. Such an integration avoids referral of a patient from one unit to another, and thus facilitates continuity of care. The planning of aftercare is of paramount importance to prevent the "revolving door" phenomenon. Such planning should always comprise an intimate collaboration with other care givers in the community, primary care, and social welfare units.

No. OF PATIENTS

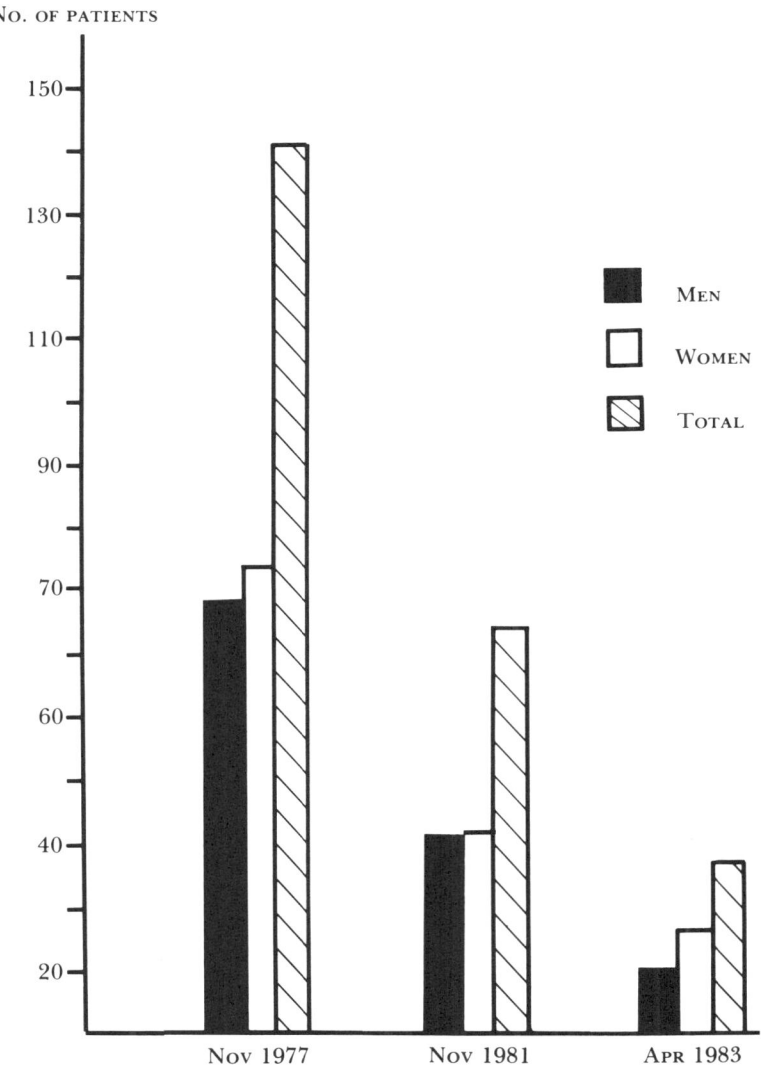

Figure 15-5.   Reduction of the long-stay patients from
the Umeå sector at the mental hospital
between 1977 and 1984.

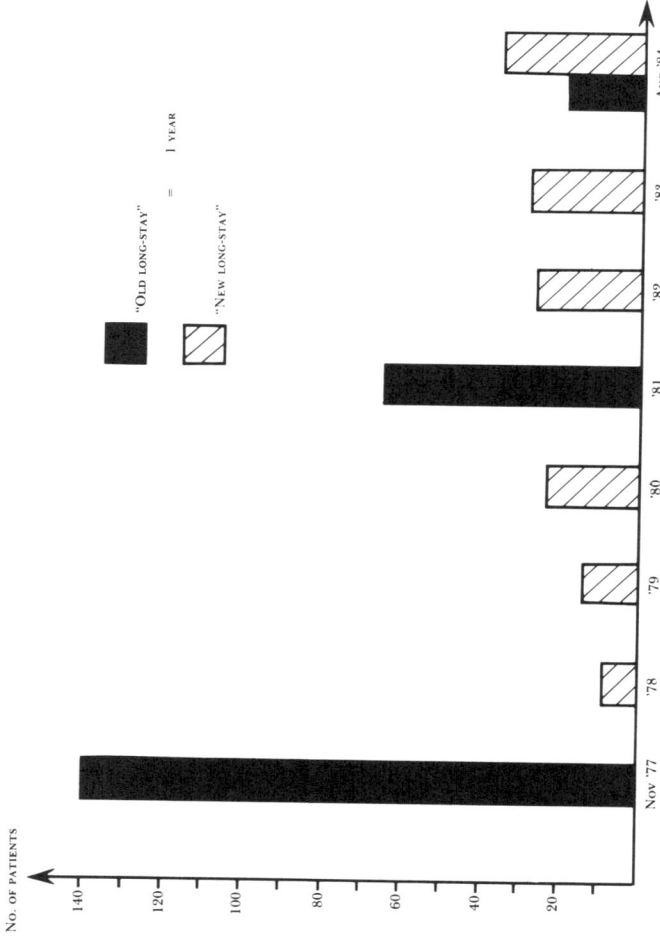

Figure 15-6. **The Umeå sector: Successive decrease of old long-stay patients at the mental hospital, and accumulation of new long- stay patients.**

REFERENCES

1. Brown, B. S. Deinstitutionalization and community support systems. Statement by the Director, National Institute of Mental Health, Rockville, MD, November 4, 1975. Mimeographed.
2. Perris, C., & Kemali, D. (Eds.). Focus on the Italian psychiatric reform. *Acta Psychiatrica Scandinavica*, Supplement 316, Vol. 71.
3. Bachrach, L. L. Deinstitutionalization: An analytical review and sociological perspective. Washington, DC: US Dept of Health, Education and Welfare (DHEW) publication no 4 (Adm) 1976, 76–351.
4. Perris, C., & Jacobsson, L. Reorganization of psychiatric services in a particular geographical area. Proceedings, 2nd International Symposium on Rehabilitation in Psychiatry, Örebro, Sweden, September 12–14, 1972.
5. Perris, C. Changing patterns of psychiatric care in Sweden. In D. Kemali, P. L. Morosini, & A. Amati (Eds.), *Servizi sanitari e psichiatrica, Obbiettivi, metodi nella pianifica e valutazione.* Roma: Il Pensiero Scientifico, 1982.
6. Perris, C., Rodhe, K., Palm, A., Hallgren, S., Lilja, C., & Söderman, H. Fully integrated in- and outpatient services in a psychiatric sector. *Social Psychiatry*, 1985, *20*, 60–69.
7. Perris, C. Community psychiatric service and aftercare of the patients returned to the community in the organization of a Swedish mental hospital. *International Journal of Social Psychiatry*, 1966, *12*, 293–298.
8. Perris, H., Hörnqvist, M., & Lundberg, S. Bedomning av livskvalitet hos avinstitutionaliserade patienter och hos patienter som fortfarande vistas på sjukhus i Västerbotten, Rep. Dept. of Psychiatry, Umeå Univ New Series No. 3, 1983.
9. Palm, U., Karlsson, K.-E. & Perris, C. Evaluation of future needs for long-stay patients in the process of deinstitutionalization. Proceedings, International Symposium on Alternatives to Institutional Care—Issues of Evaluation. Umeå, Sweden, March 15–17, 1982. SPRI Publication, 1984, 283–295.
10. Perris, C., Palm, U., Karlsson, K.-E., Perris, H., & Hornqvist, M. Omvårdnadsbehov inför avinstitutionalisering. *Nord Psykiat Tidskr*, 1984, *38*, 613–622.

Chapter 16

COPING WITH SCHIZOPHRENIA AT HOME

John K. Wing, M.D., Ph.D.

THE COURSE OF SCHIZOPHRENIA

Schizophrenia is, at one and the same time, an illness, a disability, and a way of life. The same is true of many disorders that tend to lead to long-term handicaps. The essence of coping, whether with diabetes or multiple sclerosis or blindness, is to find a way to live with the condition that avoids the accumulation of preventable impairments, social disadvantages, and personal despair, so that social disablement is minimized and the quality of life maximized.

This chapter is not concerned with that group of people who experience schizophrenia as a brief though painful episode and recover with little residual disability. According to several recent follow-up studies, this favorable outcome occurs in 20 to 25 percent of all those who are first given the diagnosis.[1-6] However, a similar proportion improves very little from the time of first onset. The remaining 50 to 60 percent of disorders run a fluctuating long-term course that can be substantially influenced by medication and by factors in the physical and psychosocial environment.

I shall briefly review the problems that living with chronic schizophrenia raises for the afflicted person and the family and suggest how some of them can be prevented and others relieved. A more detailed account of the research underlying these views can be found elsewhere.[7-10] Some of the points made may seem elementary to professional readers but I have tried to view schizophrenia through the eyes of the relatives. It is an instructive exercise. All professionals should undertake it before they consider themselves qualified to give advice.

PROBLEMS AS SEEN BY THE FAMILY

Several family problems emerge at once from a study of the statistics of the course. First admission and first-ever contact rates (the latter calculated from case registers) show that onset occurs earlier in men than women. It is not surprising therefore that men more often remain single and stay in the parental household. Women are more often married but the divorce and separation rate is high.

A study of schizophrenic patients admitted to three English mental hospitals in 1956 showed that, on discharge, 40 percent went to live with parents, 37 percent (mostly women) with a spouse, 8 percent with some other relative or friend, and 15 percent went to lodgings, rooming houses, or residential jobs. By the time of follow-up, 5 years later, only 29 percent were living with parents; there was less change in the other groups. Few separations from parental homes were due to disturbed behavior, which parents tolerated with remarkable fortitude. A third were due to the death or ill-health of a parent and a third to constructive reasons for leaving. Parents often made very little complaint even why they felt great distress, and some developed very skillful methods of managing disturbed behavior. Three-quarters of the parents were over the age of sixty and 40 percent over the age of seventy.[3]

There was a high divorce and separation rate, probably three times that in the general population. It was particularly high among men. Although a much smaller proportion of the men had married, the rate of separation was nearly double that

of the women. Disturbed behavior was responsible for nearly all
the separations during the follow-up period. Other studies have
emphasized the difference in the types of social problem experienced by parents and spouses. If neighbors come to call, it
is fairly socially acceptable for a mother to say that her son is
sick, by way of explanation of the fact that he dashed for the
safety of his room as soon as he hears the doorbell ring, and
does not come down until the visitors have gone. Such behavior
by a husband or wife is much more difficult for the partner to
explain, particularly if there are children about.[11-14] On the
whole, it is the female relative who carries most of the burden,
whatever the degree of relationship.

As the time goes on, there is no doubt that patient and relative, if they stay together, come to acquire a tolerance which
neither might have had earlier. The relative, however, does so
at the expense of restricting his or her life. Often the parents
of unmarried schizophrenics are elderly widows who are glad
to have some companionship, to have someone to do a bit of
shopping if they are physically disabled, and who are not too
worried at not being able to live a life of their own. Under such
circumstances, even a patient with a turbulent history of frequent breakdowns may eventually settle into a routine. It is another kind of institutionalism, less expensive, of course, and less
demanding of the patient than a good hospital with workshops,
leisure activities, and socialization programs would be, and
sometimes a good deal more restricting on the activities and in-
terests of relatives. Few, however, in those days, complained.
The major problem raised by relatives articulate enough to be
able to make a point is worry over the patient's future. One
father called it the WIAG ("when I am gone") syndrome.[15]

However, this contented, if restricted, outcome for family
life, at least for the unmarried patient, is sometimes only
reached after what is, in some cases, a lengthy and profoundly
distressing time, during which the patient's condition is con-
stantly unstable and the relatives do not know what will happen
next. It is not surprising that many patients find themselves
homeless and drift to common lodging houses or reception
centers. There do not have to be very many patients from each

area each year to account for the large numbers found in Salvation Army hostels and shelters for the destitute.[16, 17]

Since relatives are almost as much on the front line as patients, so far as living with schizophrenia is concerned, it is surprising that there have been so few informed surveys of their views on the subject. Much work appears to have been carried out with the major object of selecting quotations that fit the author's preconceptions of the pathogenesis of schizophrenia. Relatives do, of course, acquire considerable experience in coping with difficult behavior but their methods are inevitably trial and error. Some learn not to argue with a deluded patient; others never learn. Some discover just how far they can go in trying to stimulate a rather slow and apathetic individual without arousing resentment. Others push too hard, find their efforts rejected or that they make matters worse, and then retreat into inactivity themselves. Some never give up intruding until the patient is driven away from home.

A recent survey of the experience of relatives was undertaken with the deliberate objective of learning from them what could be done to help people with schizophrenia. Fifty patients were living with relatives who had joined a newly formed voluntary organization, the National Schizophrenia Fellowship, and another 30 were selected from those known to specialists in an area of southeast London where services were reasonably good. The two groups therefore formed a marked contrast, since it was to be expected that relatives who joined the Fellowship would be articulate and responsible, but also that they would have particularly marked problems. Between the two groups it was possible to form a clear impression of the difficulties of families.[15]

Altogether, two-thirds of the 80 patients were reported as being markedly or somewhat underactive. However, even those who had some activity tended to adopt some ritual way of spending the time, for example by brewing tea continuously or chain-smoking. One relative explained graphically, "In the evenings you go into the sitting room and it's in darkness. You turn on the light, and there he is, just sitting there, staring in front of him." Some relatives used the word "uncanny" to describe this kind of behavior. One mother said her son spent most of his time closeted in his room, only coming out at night when everyone was in bed. Usually he was talking to himself, and moving about, but every few weeks there would be complete silence for a few days. "After that has been going on for a day or two, I sometimes wonder whether he is dead."

Relatives had various theories to explain the periods of total inactivity and the long hours spent in bed. Many felt that it was because ordinary everyday living and contact with people was simply an unbearable effort to the individual suffering from schizophrenia—he had to withdraw and "recharge" himself frequently. As one mother put it, "He just can't bear people—even to be in the same room as another person." One patient himself explained that he had to have the time lying on his bed that he did, because he was "all fizzing up inside." Some relatives feared that if they allowed too much underactivity, the patient would get worse, and therefore insisted that the patient should perform certain household tasks, even though they had to stay in the room with him to make sure he did them and even though the pace at which he worked was often painfully slow. Others decided this kind of thing was too exhausting. "I'd sooner not ask him to wash up," one said, "because it only means he uses cold water or forgets to use any washing-up liquid, or leaves half the food on the plates." Some people tried to keep the patients active by keeping them entertained as much as possible—taking them out in the car, for walks, etc. But this was usually very draining emotionally.

About a third of the patients had odd ideas of various kinds—for example, that the neighbors were plotting against them or that some particular relative was at fault. The latter could be very distressing for the relative concerned. The odd ideas often concerned agencies or organizations whom the patient believed to have power over him or to be planning to harm him. Relatives found it difficult to know what to do when a patient expressed this kind of idea. If he said he had just been pursued up the road by a secret agent, ought they to accept what he said and pretend to believe it, or should they tell him he was imagining it? Many relatives feared that if they used the former approach they were encouraging the patient to lose touch with reality even further. But if they took the latter course, would the patient lose his confidence in them?

Patients tended to develop sudden irrational fears. They might, for instance, become fearful of a particular room in the house. Maybe they would tell the family the reason for their fear. "There's a poisonous gas leaking into that room," or "There are snakes under the bed in that room." At first relatives are baffled by this. Some admitted they had grown frustrated with a patient's absolute refusal to abandon some idea, despite all their attempts to reason with him, and had lost their temper. But they found this only resulted in the patient becoming very upset, and in any case the idea continued to be held with as much conviction as ever.

Several patients talked or laughed to themselves, but did this only in their own rooms, and not in front of their family. "If you stand outside his room you can hear that he's keeping up a more or less constant monologue in there." "Sometimes I hear shrieks of laughter coming from her room." Others, however, would sit throughout a meal laughing to themselves, regardless of who was there. Some would occasionally cry out in great distress in reaction to hallucinatory voices. A few relatives had been able to persuade a patient that he must not behave in this way in public. If he forgot and started to do it when others were present, a discreet reminder from the relative would silence him, or else he would go off somewhere alone until he had finished his muttering.

Innumerable examples like these could be given. One of the major complaints by relatives was that when they asked for advice from professional people as to the best way to react, they received no answer at all, or the question was simply turned back on them and their own amateur answers received with polite disdain. Perhaps their advisers had no better idea than they and were doing their best to conceal their ignorance?

A particularly important and distressing problem concerned compulsory admission to hospital. Relatives at the end of their tether and concerned for the long-term welfare of the patient are less inclined to argue the ins and outs of the civil rights issue than those who do not have to live in the situation, although I have met very few who are not distressed by the necessity. Relatives very rarely have advocate lawyers to argue their case for them.

Other difficulties concerned the administration of medication, the lack of sheltered work, the nonavailability of hostels or homes where the patients could go when the relatives needed a break, and the difficulty of obtaining welfare support when the patient was unwilling to claim it for himself. Relatives were often under strain themselves—depressed, anxious, and guilty. Sometimes there was division within the family as to the best way of proceeding. There was also the agony of not knowing what to tell the children.

It is extraordinary that so many relatives do manage to find a way of living with schizophrenia that provides the patient with a supportive and nonthreatening home. One way to help more to do so is to apply the results of research into the social reactivity of schizophrenia.

SOCIAL REACTIVITY OF SCHIZOPHRENIA SYMPTOMS

In the formulations of some early psychiatrists it was considered that chronic schizophrenic impairments (or "deterioration," as it was called) were ruthlessly progressive and that very little could be done to ameliorate the condition. We now know that this view was wrong. In fact, a certain hopelessness about the outcome was one of the reasons so many people with schizophrenia remained for long years in mental hospitals. Even in the 1930s, when modern ideas were beginning to be introduced, someone admitted for the first time with a diagnosis of schizophrenia stood only a one in three chance of being discharged within 2 years. After 2 years the chance of being discharged at all became extremely low. Nowadays only about 5 percent stay as long as a year. The significance of the very long stay was that a gradual process of institutionalism set in, during which the individual came to regard his own ability to cope outside hospital as hopeless even when, as happened quite often, the acute schizophrenic syndromes disappeared. There are still long-stay inpatients who do not wish to leave although they would probably be able to do so, given help.[18, 19]

During the 1950s and early 1960s, the social methods of helping people that had characterized the period of reform more than 100 years earlier were rediscovered and reintroduced. It was shown quite clearly that people with schizophrenia who lived in hospitals providing a good social environment were less handicapped by social withdrawal, slowness, and apathy, than those in hospitals where reform had not progressed so far. In other words, poverty of the social environment was harmful. This was not only true of hospitals, but of other places of living, including hostels, day centers, and the individual's own home.

A different kind of response to schizophrenia is social intrusiveness, the opposite of poverty of the social environment. Events which most people take in their stride may prove highly threatening to someone who is liable to develop acute schizophrenic attacks. Even promotion at work or getting engaged to be married, usually regarded as positive and rewarding events, may sometimes be experienced as increasing the pressure too much.[20] Too vigorous attempts at rehabilitation may also lead to relapse.[21, 22] Living at home with relatives who put on too much emotional pressure, or are too critical of the individual's disabilities, can have the same effect.[11, 23]

The essence of the problem for the individual with schizophrenia, therefore, is that he has to avoid two kinds of danger. On the one hand, too little social stimulation encourages social withdrawal, slowness, and apathy. On the other hand, too much social intrusion can lead to serious difficulties of communication and a recrudescence of the acute schizophrenic experiences. It is like walking a tightrope.

There is an interaction between family environment and the effect of medication. The more understanding and tolerant the family, the less medication is necessary. But the protective effect of medication will not overcome the really stressful environment, and too much withdrawal may also have to be corrected by administration of drugs.

Encouragement to take an interest in social, domestic, and vocational activities is often effective if it comes from familiar and trusted individuals and is not accompanied by too much emotional involvement. It is also important that the handicapped person retains control of the extent to which he participates, so that he does not expose himself to a level of stimulation that he experiences as painful, or at least only in carefully graduated doses. There is also the problem of communication. The appearance of the severely handicapped individual with schizophrenia may lead the observer (whether doctor, nurse, social worker, or relative) to suppose that attempts at communication are likely to be fruitless, and fewer and fewer attempts are made to reach him. This process can be self-perpetuating because of the temptation that social withdrawal holds out to the sufferer—it is so much easier to give up trying. And the risk of overdoing the attempt at communication is definitely present.

HELPING RELATIVES TO COPE

Clearly it is pointless to try to allocate blame when the end result is unsatisfactory. Professional people, relatives, and the sufferers themselves have to feel their way by trial and error, using a few principles for basic guidance. The most successful result is likely to come when professional counsel is informed and readily available, when a choice can be made from a range of comprehensive services, including day and residential settings providing shelter graded all the way from full protection (needed only briefly) to subsidized but otherwise open housing, and when the handicapped person and his relative fully understand the problem of interaction between schizophrenia and the environment.

Intervention during the early course of schizophrenia has been shown to be helpful. A controlled trial of specific education, counseling, and medication in relatives with a high level of "emotional expression" demonstrated a lower relapse rate in those so helped.[24] It is not yet clear how long this preventive effect will last or how far the techniques can be applied in the case of chronic schizophrenia.

It is clear, however, that the new emphasis, in many countries, on care of the disabled without recourse to large institutions, is likely to place extra burdens on relatives. It is very important, therefore, that the principles of good community care should be recognized and put into practice. These are geographical responsibility, a comprehensive range of services, and good organization and management, so as to provide continuity of care as needs change. The range of occupational, residential, and recreational facilities required is substantial. We are becoming aware, in the United Kingdom, that it is essential to have these facilities in place *before* any mental hospitals are closed (Social Services Committee Report, House of Commons, 1985);[25] otherwise the situation for people with schizophrenia and their relatives will be worse rather than better.

SELF-HELP FOR FAMILIES

As part of the consumer movement that has grown up in democratic countries all over the world, a number of relatives' organizations has been formed. The National Schizophrenia Fellowship in the United Kingdom was one of the first. A list of those known to me is given in the Appendix. A World Schizophrenia Fellowship has now been set up, with headquarters in Toronto, Canada.

Some of these organizations have learned to lobby governments and local health authorities effectively and to educate official, professional, and public opinion about the realities of living with schizophrenia. Relatives have had to live down the stigma, put upon them by professionals, that their poor parenting or coping had caused schizophrenia in the first place. This appalling theory is now, thankfully, in disrepute.

It is now the turn of professional caregivers to learn from those relatives who cope best and from those sufferers who are most articulate and understanding, and thus to be able to pass on this knowledge to others. It is only through a partnership that the problems of living with schizophrenia can be made tolerable.

APPENDIX

Relatives' Organizations

National Schizophrenia Fellowship,
78/79, Victoria Road,
Surbiton, Surrey.
Director, Ms Judy Weleminsky.

Schizophrenia Fellowship of Australia,
15, Cromwell Road,
South Yarra, 3141, Australia.
Dr. Margaret Leggatt.

Angehörigenvereinigung,
Hilfe für psychisch Erkrankt (HPE),
Wilhelminestrasse 130,
A-1160 Wien, Austria.
Herr Kurt Kirszen.

World Schizophrenia Fellowship,
365 Bloor St. E., Suite 1708,
Toronto, Ontario M4W 3L4,
Canada.
President, Mr. B. Jefferies.

Canadian Friends of Schizophrenics,
309, 95, Barber Greene Road,
Don Mils, Ontario, M3C-3E9,
Canada.
Mrs. Margaret Clark.

UNAFAM,
8 rue de Montyon,
75009, Paris, France
Dr. M. M. Boss.

Akationsgemeinschaft Stuttgart der
    Angehörigen psychisch Kranker,
Stuttgart Association of Relatives of the
    Mentally Ill,
Moehringer,
Landstrasse 51,
7000 Stuttgart 80, FRG.
Analiese Fischer.

New Life (Psychiatric Rehabilitation Association),
901, Hop Fat Commercial Centre,

490 492 Nathan Road,
Kowloon, Hong Kong.

Schizophrenia Association of Ireland,
4, Fitzwilliam Place,
Dublin 2.
Mr. Owen Mooney.

Enosh National Centre,
Tel Aviv POB 6254,
Code 61062, Israel.
Mrs. Chanita Rodney (Founder and Chairperson).

Zenkaren,
National Association for the Families of the
  Mentally Handicapped.
1989–19, OISO-machin,
NAKA-gun, KANAGAWA, Japan.
Mr. Takehisa Takizwa.

New Zealand Schizophrenia Fellowship,
PO Box 593, Christchurch,
New Zealand.

Dr. M. Geiser,
3011, Berne,
Kafiggasschen, 10,
Switzerland.

National Alliance for the Mentally Ill,
1901, North Fort Myer Drive,
Suite 500, Arlington,
VA 22209, USA

Schizophrenia Association of Great Britain,
International Schizophrenia Centre,
Bryn Hyfryd,
The Crescent,
Bangor, Gwynedd, LL57 2AG
Mrs. G. Hemmings, B.Sc., (Director General).

REFERENCES

1. Bleuler, M. *Die schizophrenen Geistesstörungen im Licte langjähriger Kranken und Familiengeschichte*. Stuttgart: Thieme, 1972.
2. Bleuler, M. The long-term course of schizophrenic psychoses. In L. C. Wynne, R. L. Cromwell, & S. Matthysse (Eds.) *The nature of schizophrenia*. New York: Wiley, 1978.
3. Brown, G. W., Bone, M., Dalison, B., & Wing, J. K. Schizophrenia and social care. Maudsley Monograph No. 17. London; Oxford University Press, 1966.
4. Ciompi, L. The natural history of schizophrenia in the long term. *British Journal of Psychiatry*, 1980, *136*, 413–420.
5. Ciompi, L., & Muller, C. H.: *Lebensweg und alter der schizophrenen: Eine Katemnestische langzeitstudie bis in senium*. Heidelberg; Springer, 1976.
6. Huber, G., Gross, G., & Scheuttler, R. *Schizophrenie: Eine verlaufs- und sozial—Psychiatrische langzeitstudie*. Heidelberg; Springer, 1979.
7. Wing, J. K. The management of schizophrenia in the community. In G. Usdin, (Ed.) *Psychiatric Medicine*. New York: Brunner/Mazel, 1977.
8. Wing, J. K. Social influences on the course of schizophrenia. In L. C. Wynne, R. L. Cromwell, & S. Matthyse, (Eds.) *The nature of schizophrenia*. New York: Wiley, 1978.
9. Wing, J. K. *Reasoning about Madness*. London: Oxford University Press, 1978.
10. Wing, J. K. Psychosical factors affecting the long-term course of schizophrenia. In press. (German translation to be published in 1986.)
11. Brown, G. W., Birley, J. L. T., & Wing, J. K. Influence of family life on the course of schizophrenic disorders: A replication. *British Journal of Psychiatry*, 1972, *121*, 241–258.
12. Hirsch, S. R., Gaind, R., Rohde, P. D., Stevens, B. C., & Wing, J. K. Outpatient maintenance of chronic schizophrenic patients with long-acting fluphenazine: Double blind placebo trial. *British Medical Journal*, 1973, *1*, 633–637.
13. Stevens, B. Dependence of schizophrenic patients on elderly relatives. *Psychological Medicine*, 1972, *2*, 17–32.

14. Vaughn, C. E., Patterns of interaction in families of schizophrenics. In H. Katschning, (Ed.) *Die andere Seite der Schizophrenie: Patienten zu Hause*. Vienna: Urban & Schwarzenberg, 1977.

15. Creer, C., & Wing, J. K. *Schizophrenia at home*. National Schizophrenia Fellowship, 1974.

16. Leach, J., & Wing, J. K. *Helping destitute men*. London: Tavistock, 1980.

17. Tidmarsh, D. & Wood, S. Psychiatric aspects of destitution. In J. K. Wing, & A. Hailey, (Eds.) *Evaluating a community psychiatric service*. London: Oxford University Press, 1972.

18. Wing, J. K. Institutionalism in mental hospitals. *British Journal of Clinical Social Psychology*, 1962, *1*, 38–51.

19. Wing, J. K., & Brown, G. W. *Institutionalism and schizophrenia*. London: Cambridge University Press, 1970.

20. Brown, G. W., & Birley, J. L. T. Crisis and life changes and the onset of schizophrenia. *Journal of Health and Human Behavior*, 1968, *9*, 203–214.

21. Stevens, B.: Evaluation of rehabilitation for psychotic patients in the community. *Acta Psychiatrica Scandinavica*, 1973, *49*, 169–180.

22. Wing, J. K., Bennett, D. H., & Denham, J. *The industrial rehabilitation of long-stay schizophrenic patients*. Medical Research Council Memorandum No. 42, London, H.M.S.O., 1964.

23. Vaughn, C. E., & Leff, J. P. Schizophrenia and family life. *Psychology Today*, 1976, *10*, 13–18.

24. Leff, J. P., Kuipers, L., Berkowitz, R. Eberlein-Vries, R., & Sturgeon, D.: A controlled trial of social intervention in the families of schizophrenic patients. *British Journal of Psychiatry*, 1982, *141*, 121–134.

25. Social Services Committee, House of Commons. *Community care with special reference to adult mentally ill and mentally handicapped people*. Second Report from the Social Services Committee. London: HMSO, 1985.

Chapter 17

FAMILY ATMOSPHERE ON THE COURSE OF CHRONIC SCHIZOPHRENIA TREATED IN A COMMUNITY MENTAL HEALTH CENTER

A Prospective Longitudinal Study

Michael Madianos, M.D.,
George Gournas, M.D.,
Vlassis Tomaras, M.D.,
Aphrodite Kapsali, M.D. and
Costas Stefanis, M.D.

Over the past 2 decades the study of family factors in schizophrenia have become a subject of growing interest. The relationship between family atmosphere and the course of schizophrenic psychoses has long been established.[1-4]

Certain intrafamilial communication patterns such as criticism, hostility, dissatisfaction, and emotional overinvolvement were shown to be associated with exacerbation of psychotic symptomatology and relapse of the schizophrenic patient. Along with the family emotional atmosphere, certain sociodemographic and medical variables, such as sex, marital status, previous work, and drug maintenance, were found to be not only interrelated but also relapse predictors.[5]

None of these studies have included the type of aftercare service as a mediating factor between the emotional environment and the discharged patient.

On this issue Vaughn and Leff[3] realized the need of an active intervention in high expressed emotion families, in order to regulate the number of face-to-face contacts of the patient with family members, and sometimes solving the problem of living accomodation by relocating the patient. Leff et al.[6] reported a controlled trial of social intervention in the families of schizophrenic patients in high contact with high expressed emotion relatives. One-half of the subjects were randomly assigned to routine outpatient care, while the other half received a package of social interventions. It was found that 50 percent of the patients in the routine outpatient care relapsed, compared with 9 percent in the experimental group in a 9-month period. It appears that changing the family attitudes and atmosphere is beneficial for the management of schizophrenics in the community.

The aim of the present study was to investigate prospectively the effects of a certain type of community based psychiatric aftercare on the family atmosphere and on certain indices of the illnesses course (relapses and readmission) in a cohort of 77 chronic schizophrenic patients, residents of two boroughs of greater Athens. This area is served by a Community Mental Health Center (CMHC) which is the first of this type in the country, and was established in 1979 by the University of Athens's Department of Psychiatry.[7]

This report is part of a prospective longitudinal study of 106 chronic schizophrenic patients within the frame of a WHO collaborative pilot Study Areas Project.[8]

MATERIAL AND METHOD

The Sample

The sample consisted of two cohorts of 77 chronic schizophrenic patients living with their families. It was systematically drawn from a case register for all persons in the catchment area, who had been in psychiatric inpatient care or had contacted any mental health service, except the private sector, in the census year of 1979.[9] The study subjects ranged in age from twenty-five to sixty years (mean of 40.1 years). The average duration of illness was 15.5 (± 9.0) years with a mean number 4.8 (± 4.0) of previous admissions to mental hospitals.

Procedure

The first cohort consisted of 21 patients receiving care by the CMHC (group A). The CMHC follow-up service is delivering a multidimensional program including drug maintenance, supportive psychotherapy, and in some cases, sociotherapy. Collaboration with the patient's family key members is an integral part of the aftercare planning and the follow-up of the patient. The family was instructed to recognize psychopathologic symptoms and was informed about the need for medication. In many cases a social worker or a psychiatrist had been visiting the families of the patient in order to solve a crisis and help the family members to cope with the patient. This approach was adopted as a regular procedure for every family with a psychotic member referred to CMHC services.

The second cohort included 56 patients with the same diagnosis, sociodemographic, economic, and clinical characteristics receiving routine outpatient psychiatric care, delivered outside the catchment area and consisting mainly of drug prescription with no family contacts (group B). Both groups were not randomly allocated, but self-selected.

The average follow-up period was 54 months. The study was prospective-longitudinal with one initial and two consecutive assessments. It was initiated between October 1979 – December 1980. The first assessment took place in May 1982 and the second in May 1984. Patients were diagnosed according to DSM III criteria for chronic schizophrenia prior to their inclusion in the study. A reliability study was designed to test the degree of agreement between the diagnoses given by the therapist, and an independent rater. The level of agreement was found to be significant.[10]

Relapse was defined as change from a residual state of the illness to reemergence of prominent psychotic symptoms.

According to research design the major outcome variables were the overall severity of illness in terms of psychopathology and functional capacity, assessed by the use of the Global Assessment Scale,[11] the social adjustment in the community measured by the Community Adjustment Scale,[10] and the family socioemotional conditions assessed by the use of Family Atmosphere Scale (FAS). The FAS scale is an original and comprehensive rating instrument constructed by the first of authors. It records quantitative scaled judgments of the patient's family life based on information reported by the patient and family members or drawn from the rater's home visits and other sources of information.

The FAS ratings, made on four-point scales, cover six dimensions of family emotional environment, such as satisfaction of family at having the patient home, dependency, feelings about the patient being an economic burden, family attitudes towards medication, interpersonal relationships, and family organization.

The t-test was used to measure the significance of difference of means in the two cohorts. The X^2 statistic was used to test the significance of differences in levels of family atmosphere and relapses or readmissions. A Pearson product moment correlation was used to test the relationship between FAS, GAS, and CAS scores.

Analysis of variance was used to study the relationship between the FAS score and certain independent variables. The statistical analysis was made by the use of SPSS.[14] For the purpose of the scale internal consistency measurement, each item with remainder of scale was correlated; then we computed coefficient alpha (a) which is the expected correlation of the scale items drawn randomly from a hypothetical pool of relevant items with an alternative sample of items of equal number.[15]

In Table 17-1, the item remainder correlations and the alpha coefficients are shown. For both assessments, item remainder correlations have shown statistically significant coefficients, implying that the scale exhibits a significant internal consistency. The coefficient alpha in both assessments exceeded the

**Table 17-1. Coefficient Alpha and Correlation of Each
Item with Remainder of the Family Atmosphere Scale
during the First and Second Assessments**

Dimensions	First Assessment (n=73)	Second Assessment (n=59)
1 Satisfaction of family	0.79*	0.77*
2 Economic burden to the family	0.62*	0.55*
3 Dependency	0.48*	0.65*
4 Attitudes towards medication	0.78*	0.71*
5 Intrafamilial relationships (rejection or scapegoating)	0.79*	0.73*
6 Family organization (roles)	0.55*	0.67*
Coefficient alpha	0.76	0.78

* = p<0.001

minimum of 0.50; so the scale could be considered a reliable instrument to detect the family atmosphere in chronic schizophrenic patients.

In both groups, there were high product moment correlation coefficients of FAS scores in the initial and the other two assessments (r: 0.94 0.89 and 0.74 in group A and r: 0.89 0.80 and 0.76 in group B).

RESULTS

Between first and second assessment, the difference between the mean FAS scores of those patients followed by the

**Table 17-2.   Average Score of Family Atmosphere Scale
Acccording to the type of Aftercare Service
during the First and Second Assessments**

	Treated in a C.M.H.C.		Treated Outside the Catchment Area	
	1st Ass/nt	2nd Ass/nt	1st Ass/nt	2nd Ass/nt
X̄	13.66	11.10[1]	13.27	13.83[2]
SE	0.98	0.62	0.59	0.85
N	21	27	52	32

t = 2.19   df 46   P<0.05   t = 0.23   N.S.
$t_{1,2}$ = 2.57   df 57   P<0.05

C.M.H.C. services, was found to be significant at a 0.05 level
(Table 17-2).

No differences in the mean FAS scores between first and
second assessment in group B patients, were observed. However, the mean FAS score between group A and B patients at
the second assessment differed significantly.

The correlation coefficients between FAS, GAS, and CAS
scores, in both groups and assessments, were found to be significantly high at a level of 0.001, implying that social adjustment of chronic schizophrenics is related to family atmosphere
and the overall severity of illness.

To examine the interaction between the FAS score and
certain independent variables, such as the overall severity of illness (GAS), the total number of previous admissions, marital
status, family income, experience of stressful life event(s), and
type of aftercare service, an analysis of variance was applied in
the total cohort during the second assessment. The results are
shown in Table 17-3.

With the exception of the total number of previous admissions and the experience of stressful life event(s) all the other
independent variables have shown a significant main effect of
FAS score formation. It turned out that all two-way interactions
were not significant, except the income X stressful life event(s)
interaction. Table 17-4 presents the distribution of relapses and

Table 17-3.   Analysis of Variance Summary Table:
Marital Status X Total Number of Previous Admissions
X Global Assessment Scale Score X Agency of
Attendance X Income X Stressful Event on Family
Atmosphere Scale Score (Second Assessment 1984) n: 57.

Source	F	Significance
Covariates	44.347	<0.001
G.A.S. (1st Assess.)	74.302	<0.001
Total N. previous admiss.	0.380	N.S.
Main Effects	6.506	<0.001
Marital Status	5.267	<0.009
Stressful Event	0.487	N.S.
Income	9.347	<0.001
Agency of Attendance	6.953	<0.002
Two way Interactions	2.236	<0.047
Mar. Status X Stress event	1.163	N.S.
Mar. Status X Income	2.091	N.S.
Mar. Status X Agency of Att.	1.663	N.S.
Stress ev. X Income	2.517	<0.05
Stress ev. X Agency of Att.	0.851	N.S.
Income X Agency	2.127	N.S.
Explained	5.928	<0.001

readmissions, according to the Family Atmosphere Scale score levels, in the total cohort and in both assessments.

In the period between the two assessments, almost all patients with negative family atmosphere relapsed or were rehospitalized, in contrast with the low proportion of relapsed or readmitted patients with positive family emotional environment.

It is to be noted that the relapse rate of patients with positive family life decreased from 56.7 percent in the first assessment to 28 percent after a 2-year period.

Table 17-4. Relapses and Readmissions According to the Family Atmosphere Scale Score Levels (First and Second Assessments)

First Assessment (May 1982)

Family Atmosphere Scale	Relapses			Readmissions		
	Yes	No	Total	Yes	No	Total
Positive (6–11)	56.7	43.3	100.0	56.7	43.3	100.0
Disturbed (12–17)	62.5	37.5	100.0	56.2	43.8	100.0
Negative (18–24)	94.7	5.3	100.0	89.5	10.5	100.0

x^2: 15.24 df 2 P<0.001 x^2: 11.23 df 2 P<0.001

Second Assessment (May 1984)

Family Atmosphere Scale	Relapses			Readmissions		
	Yes	No	Total	Yes	No	Total
Positive (6–11)	28.0	72.0	100.0	24.0	76.0	100.0
Disturbed (12–17)	59.1	40.9	100.0	27.2	72.8	100.0
Negative (18–24)	100.0	—	100.0	80.0	20.0	100.0

x^2: 10.35 df 2 P<0.001 x^2: 10.67 df 2 P<0.001

DISCUSSION

The repeated assessments of the family atmosphere of our cohorts of chronic schizophrenic patients living with their families, in a 5-year period, provide further evidence that negative family life is related to a higher risk of relapse or readmission. In a different sociocultural context, similar findings have already been reported by other investigators.[1-6, 16]

The importance of the family life variable in Greek society as predictor of the course of mental illness has already been shown.[17, 18] In a recent study from our department by Manto-nakis et al.[19] on a total of 45 discharged schizophrenic patients who returned to their families, 29, or 64.4 percent, relapsed, within a 14-month follow-up, compared to only 25 percent of relapsed patients who lived by themselves.

In this study, however, no family intervention was pursued, and family life was not measured; thus family per se was thought to be a source of stress for the psychotic patients.

It seems that criticism and sometimes open hostility toward the patient, feelings about the patient being an economic burden, dependency, noncompliance encouraged by family members, rejection, scapegoating, and family disorganization all have a negative effect on the course of schizophrenia.

In our study, the procedure of measuring these components of intrafamilial relationship in families of schizophrenics by the administration of the Family Atmosphere Scale has proven to be reliable, with a high predictive power, and has given results similar to those of other studies.[3-5, 13]

Moreover, our hypothesis that a CMHC family intervention oriented service may be more successful in preventing relapses and maintaining chronic mental patients in the community, than a routine outpatient service oriented toward the individual, has been confirmed by the results of this study.

More specifically, the long term, over a 24-month period, psychosocial intervention in families with a chronic schizophrenic member has resulted in improvement of their relationships, with reduction of criticism and hostility. It also minimized feelings of overconcern and dependency, and increased awareness of the need for medication.

As already noted, the two study groups did not differ in FAS scores at their initial assessment. This significantly minimizes the probability of bias due to self-selection of patients attending the CMHC services.

In addition to the type of aftercare, other factors such as the overall severity of illness, the marital status, and income, were found to affect the family atmosphere. However, neither the previous number of admissions nor the number of stressful life event(s) have shown a main effect on the FAS score. The latter, when interacted with the family income, influenced the FAS score formation.

If we look closely at this finding, we can see that very low income and lack of social support, particularly in this study, intensified the uncontrolled stressful life event(s) experienced, thus influencing the emotional atmosphere in the family.

Finally, the relationship between the overall severity of illness, in terms of psychopathology and social functioning, and the family atmosphere, appears to be reciprocal.

In summary, the findings of this study provide evidence of the beneficial effect of psychosocial intervention in the microenvironment of the chronic psychotic patients. Deinstitutionalization programs aiming at discharging patients back to their families, in order to succeed, have to provide for social and emotional support of the patient's family by establishing community based services. As the present study has shown, a multidimentional approach at the community level substantially contributes to relapse prevention and to positive family atmosphere.

REFERENCES

1. Brown, C. W., Monck, E. M. Carstairs, G. M. & Wing, J. K. The influence of family life on the course of schizophrenic illness. *British Journal Preventive Social Medicine*, 1962, *16*, 55–59.

2. Brown, G. W., Birley, J. T. & Wing, J. K. Influence of family life on the course of schizophrenic disorders: A replication. *British Journal Psychiatry*, 1972, *121*, 241–258.

3. Vaughn, C. E. & Leff, J. P. The influence of family and social factors on the course of psychiatric illness. *British Journal of Psychiatry*, 1976, *129*, 125–137.

4. Vaughn, C. & Leff, J. The measurement of expressed emotion in families of psychiatric patients *British Journal of Social Clinical Psychology*, 1976, *15*, 157–165.

5. Vaughn, C., Snyder, K., Freeman, W., Jones, S., Falloon, J., & Liberman, R. P. Family factors in schizophrenic relapse: A replication. *Schizophrenia Bulletin*, 1982, *3*, 425–426.

6. Leff, J., Kuipers, L., Berkowitz, R., Eberlein-Vries, R., & Sturgeon, D. A controlled trial of social intervention in the families of schizophrenic patients. *British Journal Psychiatry*, 1982, *141*, 121–134.

7. Madianos, M., & Stefanis, C. Developmental issues and interven-

tion strategies in a community Mental Health Center in Greece. In V. Hudolin (Ed.) *Social Psychiatry*, New York: Plenum, 1984.

8. Freeman, H., Fryers, T. & Henderson, J. Mental health services in Europe: 10 years after World Health Organization Regional Office for Europe Copenhagen, 1985.

9. Madianos, M., Stefanis, C., Madianou, D., & Tomaras, V. Prevalence of mental disorders and utilization of mental health services in two areas of Greater Athens. Paper presented at the WPA section of Psychiatric Epidemiology and Community Psychiatry Symposium, Edinburgh Scotland, 1985.

10. Madianos, M. The prognosis of chronic schizophrenic disorders in the community: A prospective longitudinal study (1979–1984). Associate professorship thesis, University of Athens, 1984 (in Greek).

11. Endicott, J., Spitzer, R., Fleiss, J., & Cohen, J. The Global Assessment Scale: A procedure for measuring overall severity of psychiatric disturbance. *Archives General Psychiatry*, 1976, *33*, 766, 771.

12. Spitzer, R., Gibbon, M., & Endicott, J. Family evaluation form. New York Psychiatric Institute, 1971.

13. Pais Kapur, R. L. The burden on the family of a psychiatric patient: Development on an interview schedule. *British Journal Psychiatry*, 1981, *138*, 332–335.

14. Nie, N. H., Hull, C. H., Jekins, J. C., Steinbrenner, K., & Bent, D. H. *Statistical package for the social sciences*. 1975. McGraw Hill, New York.

15. Nunnally, J. C. *Psychometric theory*. New York: McGraw Hill, 1967.

16. Barrowclough, C., Tarrier, N. Psychosocial interventions with families and their effects on the course of schizophrenia: A review. *Psychological Medicine*, 1984, *14*, 629–642.

17. Alevisatos, G., & Lyketsos, G. A preliminary report of research concerning the attitude of the families of hospitalized mental patients. *International Journal Social Psychiatry*. 1964, *10*, 37–44.

18. Safilios, Rothschild C. Deviance and mental illness in the Greek family. *Family Process*, 1968, *7*, 100–117.

19. Mantonakis, J., Jemos, J., Christodoulou, G., & Lykouras, E. Short-term social prognosis of schizophrenia *Acta Psychiatrica Scandavica*, 1982, *66*, 306–310.

Chapter 18

DEINSTITUTIONALIZATION

Alternatives to Mental Hospitals in Italy.

Eugenio Torre, M.D.

Since the end of World War II widespread opinion has held that it would be better to transfer the functions of mental hospitals to psychiatric units in general hospitals and to local nonresidential or semiresidential services. Many efforts have been directed toward carrying out this goal, but until 1978 no legislation was passed prohibiting admissions to the traditional freestanding mental hospital. In 1978 laws were passed in Italy prohibiting the admission of patients to traditional mental hospitals. Because of this change, politicians and research workers of many countries have been greatly concerned about the ongoing organization of mental health services.

In the middle of the nineteenth century there were about 60 psychiatric institutions in Italy; most of them had been built between the end of eighteenth and the beginning of the nineteenth century, and about two-thirds of them were private hospitals, often administratively run by religious organizations. Between 1861 and 1904 (establishment of the Kingdom of Italy and date of the first psychiatric Act, respectively) about 30 new psychiatric hospitals were opened; at the start of World War I there were 59 public mental hospitals (three of them were judicial hospitals) and 30 private institutions. Between 1919 and 1978 only 10 new hospitals have been built.

Since 1970 there have been many changes in the pattern of psychiatric patient care. At the beginning of the 1970s, policy was oriented toward deinstitutionalization and resettlement of patients in the community; until 1975 the situation was realistic, and the average duration of hospital stay for new patients gradually shortened and many long-stay patients were rehabilitated to their homes or, frequently, the elderly were placed in nursing homes. After 1975, providing alternative allocations for the remaining long-stay inpatients became more and more difficult, and the decrease in total inpatient population slowed down. In May 1978 a new law was enacted, the essential features of the reform being: since the date of the new act no "first ever" has been admitted to a mental hospital as an inpatient; since July 1980 in our catchment area, and in many other regions of the country, readmissions have also been prohibited; all residential treatments, both compulsory and voluntary, have been undertaken in small psychiatric wards attached to general hospitals; these units have been established with an approximative ratio of 0.15 beds per 1000 population. And it has been suggested that the greater part of long- and short-term care should be assigned to outpatient departments; and local health authorities have been invited to provide the resources for non-residential services.

Although Italian mental hospitals are closed to new admissions, some long-stay patients, mostly suffering from functional psychoses, continue to live in the traditional hospitals. The construction of new large mental hospitals is prohibited; these changes have resulted in a marked reduction in the number of beds for residential treatments, especially for those patients needing more than 2 or 3 months of hospitalization; there are very few alternative settings for long-term care. There exists also a profound difference among regions and provinces, especially between the North and the South, as to the phasing of the deinstitutionalization program and the implementation of the new Act.

The effects of the new law have been evaluated in several studies and some results seem consistent:[1, 2] There is a reduction of compulsory admissions, easier access to outpatient services, and an increase in the care provided by professionals other than psychiatrists. In the meantime, more than five projects for modifying the law have been proposed by various parties, unions and psychiatric associations.[3] No one can guess the eventual development that will occur in the organization of Italian psychiatric services. But some trends can be described on the basis of empirical data however tentative and parochial they may be.

UTILIZATION OF SERVICES

In 1975 a psychiatric case register modeled after that in London[4, 5] was set up for a catchment area (Lomest) near Pavia in Lombardia, a region of northern Italy.[6-9] Subsequently case register procedures were set up in three additional regions of northern Italy, and comparisons of statistics were made.[10-15] Thus, information concerning the utilization of mental health services from a population of about 300,000 inhabitants, or 0.5 percent of the total Italian population, is available.

Some sociodemographic characteristics of the health areas are summarized in Table 18-1. Lomest is a medium-sized town in Lombardia; Albenga in Liguria and Novi in Piemonte are areas comprising a small town (less than 20,000 inhabitants) and many small rural villages; Sestri is a district of a large town (Genova) in Liguria. As would be expected, agricultural workers comprise about 20 to 25 percent of the population in Albenga and Novi, but are not significantly represented in the larger towns. In each area the percentage of economically active population is higher than the national mean.

The mental hospital of each area lies outside its respective zone; the general hospital psychiatric unit is located within the area itself in Sestri and Novi, but about 65 km away from Lomest and Albenga. The outpatient service for Lomest has been operating since 1975, and since 1979–1980 for the other areas.

Table 18-2 shows the prevalence rates and the distribution of various types of care provided in Lomest. The 1-year prevalence rates include four components: a) inpatients on census day (December 31 of the previous year); b) patients who make

Table 18-1. Sociodemographic Characteristics of Four Areas in Northern Italy (1871)

	Lomest	*Albenga*	*Novi*	*Sestri*
Total Population	80838	52548	77298	86187
Inhabitants/km²	486	174	105	4100
Males/Females	0.93	0.96	0.94	0.94
% Aged 0–14	20	18	17	19
% Aged 65 +	13	16	18	14
% Economically Active (Aged 15 +)	42	47	56	43
Occupation				
% Agriculture		24	18	1
% Manufacturing	2	26	50	55
% Trade and	67	50	32	44
Services	31			

contact with the hospital during the year following the census day; c) outpatients actually attending the nonresidential service before and after census day with no more than 3 months between attendances; d) patients who make contact with the outpatient department during the year following the census day. The table reveals that the overall rates increased until 1978, but after passage of the law they seem to level off at a rate of 8 per 1,000 population aged fifteen and over. According to different patterns of contact, the most relevant features are: Numbers of people in the hospital on census day remain fairly stable; hospital admissions are decreasing; outpatient treatment rates are about four times higher than inpatient rates.

Since the surviving old long-stay inpatients are not particularly elderly, it might be assumed that they will remain a heavy load on the psychiatric care system for a long time. The number of new long-stay inpatients cannot increase because the buildup of these patients is prohibited by the veto on admissions under the new Act. The question, however, is: Does the new law eliminate chronic long-stay inpatients? Formally, the answer is affirmative, but caution must be exercised at the substantive level. Edwards & Carter[16] have suggested that cohorts

**Table 18-2.   One-Year Prevalence (1976–1982)
for Various Type of Contact: Rates per 1000 Population Aged 15 +**

Type of Contact	1976	1977	1978	1979	1980	1981	1982
A: Inpatient on 31 Dec. of previous year	0.85	0.95	0.87	0.76	0.73	0.68	0.64
B: Not A, but admitted during the year	1.55	1.37	0.76	1.09	0.87	0.81	0.90
C: Not A and B; outpatient on 31 Dec. of previous year	1.83	2.16	1.63	1.18	2.25	2.14	1.41
D: Not A, B and C, but outpatient contact during the year	2.92	3.31	4.76	4.64	4.38	4.36	4.56
Total	7.15	7.79	8.01	7.67	8.18	7.99	7.49

of people in prolonged contact with day services are building up more and more. Presumably in Lomest there is also an increase in high-user groups of patients attending nonresidential services, and they will not differ significantly from the new long-stay inpatients who accumulated before the 1978 Act.

The closure of large traditional mental hospitals seems to have produced a drop in admission rates (less than one per 1,000) and this may principally concern those who are not mentally ill but only homeless and in need of food. The trend may be an effect of the marked reduction in the number of beds; we do not believe that a ratio of about 0.15 beds per 1,000 population is realistic for the satisfaction of residential treatment needs of the mentally ill unless a very extended network of outpatient care has been previously set up. At present, this is not the case in Italy; sometimes more bed availability is obtained by utilizing the "revolving door technique"; sometimes patients receive diversified treatment or are allocated to nonpsychiatric residences. The danger is that some patients drop out of care or that the waiting list on other wards grows longer.

Treated outpatients tend to increase and, more and more, they seem to be young men and middle-aged women; at present time, it is difficult to say whether this trend expresses temporal changes in a particular diagnostic category or a change in referral habits among general practitioners. Outpatients in treatment seem to be composed of two large categories: people who remain patients in contact with the conventional clinics for prolonged periods of time and those who terminate treatment after a few visits. The former are for the most part discharged psychotics; the latter seem to be people suffering essentially from minor psychiatric disorders. The high-user patients represent only about 20 percent of the total 1-year prevalence rates, but account for about 80 percent of the total service activities; if this trend is verified in replicated evaluative studies, it will suggest a danger that the nonresidential psychiatric facilities will be restricted to the specific function of care givers for chronic patients suffering from those mental disorders that produce the most serious impairments.

Figure 18-1 shows the distribution of contacts in four areas

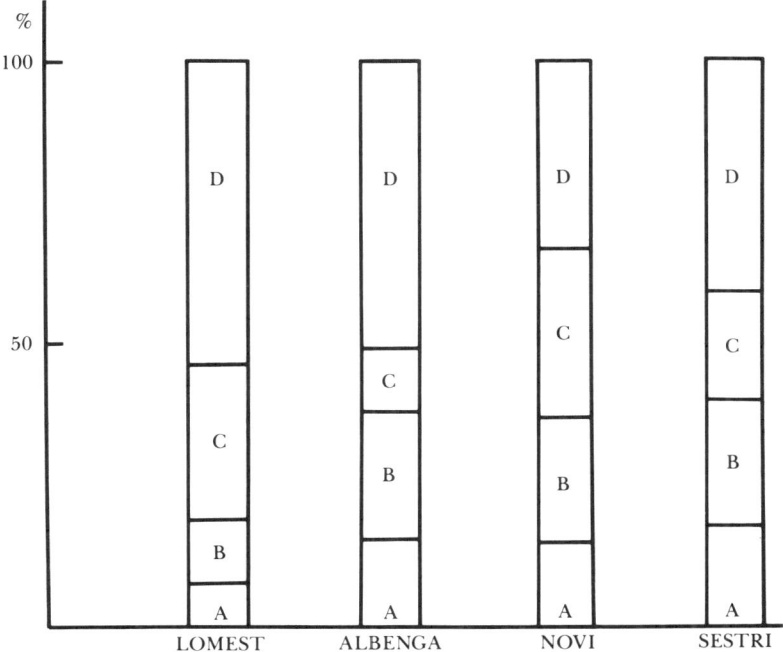

**Figure 18-1.   Total patient population (1981) in four
areas by types of contact with in-and
outpatient facilities: Percentage (A, B, C,
D as in Table 18-2).**

of Northern Italy. There are similarities and differences but the
former seem to outnumber the latter; however, the trends are
not homogeneous everywhere. Average estimates from different areas are somewhat confusing because of the influence of
additional factors probably contributing to various distributions
within the areas involved. Some of the factors may include a
different impact of the deinstitutionalization program, sociodemographic characteristics of the zones, the distance from residential settings, and the more or less community-oriented policy of the services. The relative weight of these factors upon

different distributions of care might be an issue for further research, both in general and specifically for patients suffering from fuctional psychoses needing long-term treatment. In this respect, collaborative projects among different countries might produce useful information for the more rational utilization of new resources, even though the actual allocation of money to health care services does not seem a first priority of many governments.

Table 18-3 presents the annual rates of "new on the register" patients from 1976 to 1982; they had never been admitted to public mental hospitals, but it was possible that they had been cared for in private institutions before 1976. Admissions sharply decreased in 1978, after which time they seemed to level off at a rate of 0.1 to 0.2 per 1,000 population; new contacts with outpatient services were apparently stable both before and after the 1978 law. These figures however, are, rather crude and it would be a mistake to place too much confidence in them. It will be necessary to devise a detailed study to separate the real "new" patients from those who are "new" only because previous contacts are unknown. Nevertheless, because the examined population is relatively stable, it would not be too arbitrary to assume that the calculated rates were not overly biased.

Hence, the question arises as to where and how patients needing long-term treatment will accumulate after the closing of hospitals. A preliminary answer may be based on four sets of data that refer to the buildup of high-user patients in the services. Obviously, the definition of these patients is arbitrary, and therefore operational statements have been tentatively investigated.

(1) The high-user group of outpatients are those who were in continuous contact with the outpatient department for 1 year or more, with a maximum period of 3 months between attendances. Between 1976 and 1978, 762 patients were recorded on the Lomest case register list; of these patients, 69 satisfied the established criteria. Almost all of them were patients previously discharged from the hospital; two out of three were classified as suffering from schizophrenia or affective psychoses. It seems that before the new reform, about 10 percent of the patients utilizing mental health services became people in prolonged contact with the conventional outpatient clinics. In the mean-

Table 18-3. One-Year Incidence:
Rates per 1000 Population Aged 15 +

Year	Inpatients	Outpatients	Total
1976	.69	2.24	2.93
1977	.54	1.91	2.45
1978	.09	2.15	2.24
1979	.22	1.96	2.18
1980	.15	2.00	2.15
1981	.17	1.39	1.56
1982	.23	1.85	2.08

time, another type of accumulation was in progress in the hospital, that is, new long-stay patients.

(2) During 1977, 182 "new on the register" patients were recorded from Lomest, and of these patients, 55 were classified as suffering from functional psychoses. A 4-year follow-up study was carried out and the high-user group of patients were those who, at no more than 3-month intervals, made frequent visits to the outpatient clinics and occasionally were admitted to the hospital, usually to the small ward within the general hospital. Of the 55 psychotic patients, 50 percent were in continuous long-term care during the 4 years following their first contact with the services, but 30 percent disappeared after one or two contacts, even though clinical conditions were similar.

(3) In 1976 the 1-year prevalence rate of schizophrenics from Lomest was 1.87 per 1,000 population aged fifteen and over (Table 18-4); 121 patients were involved in this group. Between 1977 and 1981, 57 new cases of schizophrenia were recorded on the register. In 1981 the rate was 1.93 and number 125. Of these patients 81 had been previously registered in 1976; further, in 1981, 40 of the 1976 cohort, plus 13 from the 57 new cases accumulated between 1977 and 1981, made up those not in treatment. These data seem a good replication of the previous studies; indeed, more than 50 percent of the patients became chronic users of the services and about 30 percent quickly dropped out of care.

(4) A follow-up study was set up for investigating differences, if any, between groups of patients who became high-user

Table 18-4.   Schizophrenic Patients from Lomest.
One-Year Prevalence (1976–1981) for Various
Types of Contact: Rates per 100,000 Population
Aged 15 + (A, B, C, D as in Table 18-2)

	1976	1977	1978	1979	1980	1981
A	40	37	43	40	42	40
B	54	56	34	48	48	38
C	60	62	42	25	59	64
D	33	36	68	73	59	51
Total	187	191	187	186	208	193

attenders of psychiatric services in two periods of time, one before and one after the new Italian reform. One hundred ninety-
six patients in care on 31 December 1976 and 160 in care on 31
December 1980 were followed up during 1977 and 1981 respectively. After 1 year the two cohorts were divided into low-
and high-user patients according to whether or not they met the
further criteria of 1 year in continuous contact (no gap longer
than 3 months) with services during the year following the census day. The more relevant results seem to be that the patient
group was markedly older than the general population in both
years and that the patient cohorts differed, the 1976 series having practically no subject in the youngest age group and the
1980 series having the highest percentage in the oldest age
group. This higher number of patients in the youngest group
was probably due to an easier access to the community services
after the 1978 reorganization of the psychiatric care system.
Furthermore, women were more represented in both cohorts
and the ratio differed significantly from that of the general
population; the surplus of women increased in the oldest age
group and the figure can presumably be accounted for by sex
differences in mortality. High-user patients were likely to be
single rather than married, and sex differences with regard to
marital status were not significant in any age group. The Lomest-born people were 73 percent of the total general population according to 1981 census; the distribution of the high-user

patients with respect to place of birth revealed that the Lomest-born patients represented only one out of three subjects in both series.

FURTHER RESEARCH

Usually, to raise new a issue is a fascinating task, but to establish priorities is more difficult, and to select between empirical projects involves even heavier responsibility. Therefore, I will suggest just three questions that are starting points for surveys in progress or might become aims of future collaborative studies.

There are indications that severely psychotic patients, after their first contact with services, split into two groups: those who become patients in prolonged contact[16, 17] and those who disappear after a few attendances; but to say a priori who will become a member of which category is hazardous. Is it possible at the first assessment to discriminate between the two? Are there reliable criteria of assessment and outcome? Is it possible to plan collaborative follow-up studies on this issue in order to minimize costs and permit small, financially limited research groups to face the problem?

There is a good deal of information about relationships between long-stay periods in the hospital and institutionalism, and there are some indications that high-user groups of patients show symptoms of high dependency on new residential and nonresidential psychiatric settings. Is it possible to modify assessment methods for the old institutionalism into new procedures more fitting the characteristics of the new dependency?

The opening of nonresidential psychiatric services and their closeness to the patient's home provide easier access to the various levels of care.[18] As a consequence of this, there are indications that some severely psychotic chronic patients living at home outside the network of care and having social contacts exclusively with their relatives, now feel drawn to psychiatric services. From a certain point of view, they may be considered as people suffering from institutionalism but outside psychiatric institutional facilities. It would be useful to verify if these types of patients are few and accidental, or if they represent a consistent subgroup of chronic psychotics. In the latter case, it would be valuable to learn from the patients and their relatives what means they devised for coping with the effects of the psychosis without assistance from the psychiatrist.

CONCLUSION

Many additional studies are needed before an overall judgment can be made as to whether or not the Italian Act has produced any progress toward a development of truly community based mental health services. Some tentative indications may be discussed.

In the near future, where available, resources will probably be invested in residential structures for medium-term care as alternatives to the old mental hospitals. Organizational aspects are relevant but they are not the only issues to be considered; adequate patient assessment, evaluation of clinical and social outcomes, and the adaptation of patterns of care designed to meet the specific needs of individual patients must become the ultimate goals of each new facility. It is obvious that health planners must accept constant monitoring and evaluative research as essential features of any service innovation. Unfortunately, administrators continue to evade these necessities, at least in our country.

If available data are consistent, they seem to indicate that the treatment of minor psychiatric disorders is the Cinderella of public mental health service activities. In fact, however, if neurotic patients need only drugs, then family doctors are sufficient to prescribe and followup on these cases. If they need more sophisticated psychotherapeutic treatments, public clinics do not seem an appropriate setting in which to care for them. The danger is in the development of a system of public health services for the more severely mentally ill, while private practice serves the needs of people suffering minor psychiatric disorders. It is easy to predict that a strict selection based on socioeconomic status of the patients will develop. Therefore, devising methods of care to cater to the needs of patients suffering from minor psychiatric disorders should become a more relevant concern of people involved in the public mental health system.

Our studies suggest the considerable need for research policy which will be able to provide scientific conclusions and pragmatic indications for the kind of mental health services that meet the needs of the patient population.

REFERENCES

1. Tansella, M., Meneghelli, G., & Siciliani, O. Implementing a community psychiatric service in South Verona under the new Italian mental health act. *Psychiatric Social Science*, 1982, *2*, 105–111.
2. Misiti, R. Future developments in Italy. Presented at the ESF workshop on Needed areas of research on long-term treatment on functional psychoses, Bagnaia, Italy, May 9–11, 1983.
3. FCRS sulla Devianza e emarginazione: Manicomiomania, testi delle proposte di legge sulla 180. Ed.Dedalo, Bari, 1982.
4. Wing, L., Branley, C., Hailey, A. M., & Wing, J. K. Camberwell cumulative psychiatric case register, Part I. Aims and methods. *Social Psychiatry*, 1968, *3*, 116–121.
5. Wing, J. K., Hailey, A. M. (Eds.): *Evaluating a community psychiatric service: The Camberwell Register 1964–71*. Nuffield Provincial Hospitals Trust. London: Oxford University Press, 1972.
6. Torre, E., Marinoni, A., & Allegri, G. Lomest psychiatric case register: Old and new long-stay patients. *Social Psychiatry*, 1982, *17*, 130–136.
7. Torre, E., Marinoni, A., Allegri, G., Bosso, A., Ebbli, D., & Gorrini, M. Trends in admissions before and after an Act abolishing mental hospitals: A survey in three areas of northern Italy. *Comprehensive Psychiatry*, 1982, *23*, 211–216.
8. Marinoni, A., Torre, E., Allegri, G., & Comelli, M. Lomest psychiatric case register: The statistical context required for planning. *Acta Psychiatrica Scandinavica*, 1983, *67*, 109–117.
9. Marinoni, A., Torre, E., & Comelli, M. Evaluating mental health services in Italy. *The Statistician*, 1985, *34*, 25–29.
10. Torre, E., Ebbli, D., Marinoni, A., Allegri, G., Ciancaglini, P., & Castelnovi, C. I registri dei casi psichiatrici di Lomest e dell'Al-

benganese: Confronto di dati per la valutazione dei servizi. *Rivista Sperimentale di Freniatria*, 1983, *107*, 62–78.

11. Torre, E., Marinoni, A., Girardengo, C., Scoglia, G., Oberti, I., & DeMicheli, V. Uno studio comparativo dell'utenza di due aree sanitarie: I registri di Lomest e del Novese. *Formazione Psichiatria*, 1983, *3*, 95–108.

12. Ebbli, D., & Bonizzoni, P. Prime valutazioni dei servizi psichiatrici di due aree sanitarie della regione Liguria: l'Albenganese e Genova I. *Formazione Psichiatria*, 1983, *3*, 129–134.

13. Girardengo, C., Giacobbe, P., & Torre, E. Il registro dei casi psichiatrici dell'Ovadese: Uno studio valutativo. *Unità Sanitaria*, 1984, *14*, 25–30.

14. Torre, E., & Marinoni, A. Evaluating community mental health services in Italy after the closing of mental hospitals. *American Journal of Social Psychiatry*, 1985, *5*, 94–98.

15. Torre, E., & Marinoni, A. Register studies: Data from four areas in northern Italy. *Acta Psychiatrica Scandinavica*, 1985, Supplement 316, *71*, 87–95.

16. Edwards, C., & Carter, J. Day services and mentally ill. In J. K. Wing, & E. Olsen (Eds.) *Community care for mentally disabled*. Oxford: Oxford University Press, 1978.

17. Sturt, E., Wikes, T., & Creer, C. A survey of long-term users of the community psychiatric services in Camberwell. In J. K. Wing (Ed.) Long-term community care: Experience in a London borough. *Psychological Medicine*, Monograph Supplement 2, 1982.

18. Keane, P. & Fahy, T. J. Who receives aftercare? Utilization of services by discharged inpatients. *Psychological Medicine*, 1982, *12*, 891–902.

Chapter 19

MENTAL HEALTH SERVICES IN GRONINGEN AND TRIESTE

Robert Giel, M.D. and
Sineke ten Horn, Ph.D.

The foreign visitor guided along mental health services in the Netherlands will be impressed by their number and differentiation: special hospitals for various categories of patients, among whom mentally disturbed offenders are those best cared for; a wide variety of outpatient services with a whole range of psychotherapeutic skills; and different types of sheltered homes for people who are disabled rather than still actively ill. Yet our evaluative studies since the mid-1970s, particularly those with our national and local registers, have revealed the deficiencies in the system—or rather, the lack of any system in the network as a whole. A few of such deficiencies are:

- no proper delineation of the catchment areas of various services, and of their resulting responsibilities towards the population;
- tremendous organizational fragmentation of the network, resulting in lack of continuity of care;
- inflexible intake or admission procedures suiting the ideology of the service rather than the needs of the population.

These problems have brought considerable criticism from the consumer organizations, the media, and parliament, and stimulated interest in alternative models of care. It is for this reason that developments in Italy for a time were quite popular in the Netherlands. The department of social psychiatry of the University of Groningen shared this interest, mainly because of our participation in the European study of Mental Health Services in Pilot Study Areas, which was coordinated by the WHO European Regional Office in Copenhagen. This study of many years' duration enables us to assess the situation in Trieste, one of the pilot areas, through visits and through a cohort study which was completed in 1982. In this chapter we want to sketch the present situation in Trieste and compare it briefly with that in the Netherlands.

During our last visit to Trieste, early in spring of 1984, the excitement inherent in democratic psychiatry seemed to have died down. Instead we could perceive disquiet about imminent changes in the famous Law 180 which decreed the closure of all mental hospitals. Revision of this law would lead to the reinstatement of hospitals, this time as rehabilitation centers for certified patients and for patients from psychiatric units in general hospitals who could not be discharged within 1 month. Beds would number one per 10,000 of the population. People appeared to agree that Law 180 in 1978 was hurried through parliament to prevent a referendum; and that it is too sketchy with regard to indications for the financial structure of the new system and for alternative services. However, proponents of Law 180 fear that its principles will be abandoned, and hope for a meaningful revision. Our experience will illustrate that reinstatement of the mental hospital could threaten the principles of democratic psychiatry, and could at best create a situation prevailing in Holland.

MENTAL HEALTH CARE IN TRIESTE

The formal mental hospital in Trieste, San Giovanni, looks dilapidated and overgrown. The 240 remaining guests form a strange assemblage, waited upon by 70 nurses and a few social workers and psychologists, according to their specific needs. For example, six nurses are available round the clock to assist a lobotomized woman. Others need no assistance. In front of the chapel, children of the staff are playing. They spend the day in the kindergarten, which is now part of the hospital.

In one of the wards we are shown the individual banking accounts of the guests; they furnish the place from their own savings. During the nights no one is on duty. Two telephone lines connect the ward with the emergency unit in the general hospital, which is staffed round the clock by two psychiatrists. On the ward, no one is in charge. According to our guide, a middle-aged male nurse, himself still in the traditional white nurse's garb, assigning such responsibility to someone would only lead to monarchism. This somewhat paternalistic person impresses us as a relic of the old days. San Giovanni has more of the air of a monument commemorating the liberation of the psychiatric patient than of a busy guesthouse.

We are to see democratic psychiatry in action in two of the seven *centri di salute mentale* serving the 290,000 inhabitants of the province of Trieste. Approximately 23 psychiatrists (8/100,000), a few psychologists and sociologists, 5 social workers, 300 nurses (1/1000) and more than 80 volunteers staff the network of facilities.

What does such a center look like? It is a large old house, open to the public from 8 a.m. to 8 p.m. for an outpatient appointment, for a meal, just to sit, or for some improvised activities. Two nurses are on duty during the nights, and are in charge of the 4 to 12 beds occupied by people admitted either from the general hospital or from one of the several apartments belonging to each center, in case they cannot maintain themselves any longer in such a place.

The seven centers have 44 beds (.15/1000), and 21 apartments lodging a total of 100 people (.34/1000; approx. .5/1000 places). Each center, with a catchment area of 25,000-45,000 people, has at least 2 psychiatrists, of whom one is on the move almost the whole day. At night two psychiatrists man the emergency unit in the general hospital. Someone admitted there outside office hours can stay overnight only. The next morning he will be transferred to the center serving his own district. To this end the centers have vehicles available.

CENTRO AURISINA AND CENTRO BARCOLA

We are first taken to rural centro Aurisino because lunch is supposed to be good there. It appears a cheerful place; someone is accompanying a group of singing patients on a guitar. Most doors are wide open, and everywhere people can be seen sitting and talking. We are immediately taken to the kitchen, where an elderly woman scolds us for being late, and later for not being able to empty our plates which are heaped high with food. Another woman entering the kitchen to get herself a glass of water surveys the table and sees that none of us has anything to drink. Without a word she corrects that situation. Later on, when we are guided through the center, we encounter both women again. They are more or less permanent inmates.

The staff appear highly motivated and enthusiastic. Their interaction with clients, and also between the various categories of clients (outpatients, daily visitors, and inmates) is open-minded and not restricted to doctor-patient roles. This does not preclude any hierarchical order headed by the psychiatrist. When we observe that in the Netherlands the ward's nursing team has the power to obstruct admission of a patient against the will of the psychiatrist on the basis of the argument that his behavior would cause too much disturbance, the response does not touch the doctor-nurse relationship. The immediate and relevant response is: "And what about the patient?" A question which in Holland is always the referring agent's business!!

What happens to a psychotic patient in this situation? We hear the story of a thirty-nine-year-old married man, who became psychotic during a trip in the mountains. His general practitioner tried to control him during the first few days of his illness. When he did not succeed, he referred him to the center. There he was too disturbed to be treated as an outpatient. Because of his suspiciousness, it took some time to convince him to take haloperidol. Because the situation tended to get out of hand, it was decided to admit some of his relatives, in the expectation that this would bring him comfort. Instead, his behavior deteriorated further, while his relatives also started to behave as patients. They were advised to return home and stay away for the time being. His parents, however, urged him to seek help in a private clinic in Venice, which he did. However, after a few weeks he returned to Aurisina, claiming that he could not stand the clinic in Venice. At the time of our visit he was much improved, and spent part of the day with his wife and children at home. In 2 weeks' time he was expected to resume his work for half-days.

From Aurisina we drive to Barcola, which is situated within Trieste. There we soon join a group of people sitting around a table. A male and a female nurse introduce themselves; they are mainly passive listeners to what goes on. An emaciated and very sleepy young man is repeatedly urged to make a phone call to his mother, but fails to do so because he has to be shaken to stay awake. He is obviously intoxicated. Most verbose is a young man who styles himself after Elvis Presley. In fluent English he tells us that he loves marijuana and amphetamines, the latter because he is too fat. He appears tremendously satisfied with himself, to the great enjoyment of another young man with long, dirty hair and very bad teeth, who sits opposite him. When we ask the Rock type what he is doing here, he informs us that he came just for fun. Perhaps he was ill yesterday, but today he is present to assist others. Perhaps we can provide him with some marijuana, because he thinks that in Holland it is free and available. Suddenly, he returns the question, asking us what we think could be wrong with him. Our response that "maybe his problem is exaggeration," causes great hilarity. The long-haired boy shows us around the center. When alone, he appears quite shy. Barcola is rather like Aurisina, perhaps more noisy and less cozy. In one of the rooms a man lies on his back on the floor, with his feet on a chair. His position looks quite uncomfortable, but he smiles at us, while keeping on his earphones which are plugged into a blasting portable radio. Our guide discloses that this man is a freak, well-known around the town.

Our guide himself lives with a friend in town. He had a girlfriend and holds a part-time job. His friend gave him the address of the center. He comes here for assistance only or to help others, because he likes the atmosphere.

Downstairs, in the corridor, there is new action. A pale middle-aged woman, who looks somewhat out of place in this context, complains in a tearful voice that she wants to go home. However, one of the nurses points out to her that she knows that she has to wait for her husband who will fetch her home. Did not she phone already, to find out that her husband was not in yet? Elvis Presley involves himself, talking loudly to the woman. The nurse informs us that the woman is depressed. We leave after saying goodbye to everyone. Outside, the sociologist accompanying us admits that compared to Aurisina, Barcola is both home and the street.

THE WHO STUDY OF MENTAL HEALTH SERVICES IN PILOT STUDY AREAS IN EUROPE

This sketch of mental health care in Trieste perhaps resembles one of the disorderly domestic scenes painted by the seventeenth century Dutch painter Jan Steen. We were of course very much interested in comparing mental health care in Trieste and Groningen. The WHO Study of Mental Health Services in Pilot Study Areas in Europe enables us to do so. The participants from Trieste had, during the more than 10 years this study took, always been somewhat averse to quantitative studies of patients contacting the services. They had more interest in telling the stories of individual patients affected by the changes in Trieste. Finally, however, they consented to a cohort study of adults contacting the services for the first time or for a new episode of illness. Patients were followed for a period of 2 years. We would like to present some of the results, which in our view show that in Trieste people seem to have achieved what they hoped, certainly when compared with the situation in Groningen.

We collected the Groningen cohort with our local case register. It consisted of 200 consecutive patients entered into the register in 1979. They were without any contact during the previous 6 months. The cohort from Trieste was collected according to the same criteria in 1980. A few psychiatrists in private practice and the 40 beds of the university department of psychiatry in the town did not participate. This unit has 800 admissions annually from a much wider area than the pilot study area. According to the investigators from Trieste, these include few people from Trieste itself. Nevertheless, it is possible that the average number of inpatient days presented in Table 19-1 is underestimating the intramural experience of the cohort from Trieste. Notwithstanding this, there are marked differences in the care delivered to the two cohorts:

1. In Trieste the average number of intramural days is less than in Groningen for each diagnostic group, both in the first and the second year of follow-up.
2. The average number of outpatient contacts and days in day care is much greater in Trieste, both during the first and the second year.

Although the Table tells us nothing about the quality nor the outcome of care, it certainly shows us the shift from inpatient to outpatient care in Trieste, which is greatly desired in the Netherlands, but has not been achieved notwithstanding the extra resources put into extramural services since the mid-1970s.

SOME CONSIDERATIONS AND CONCLUSIONS

What we encountered in Trieste was an unprofessional attitude towards psychiatry, enthusiasm, and motivation to change the social inequality that used to be inevitable in the fate of the psychiatric patient. This attitude appeared general and enduring, and it played a role in reducing the barriers between professionals and lay people. It helped to enlist the collaboration of people from outside the profession. One of its results was a cooperative, counting 1300 members, ex-patients and other outcasts of society. It operates independently of the professionals and has access to various jobs.

The idealism of the staff does not seem to exclude realism. They are well aware of the limitations of family care, and of the

Table 19-1.   The Cohorts of Trieste (Italy) and Groningen (The Netherlands)

		Average Number Per Patient:					
		in First Year			in Second Year		
	(N)	O.P. Contacts	Days Day-Care	Days I.P.	O.P. Contacts	Days Day-Care	Days I.P.
Neurosis and Personality Disorders							
T	(50)	5,9	4,7	6,2	3,3	1,3	0,6
G	(79)	4,9	—	30,5	0,3	—	20,0
Addictions							
T	(32)	13,1	8,7	1,7	7,8	4,0	2,6
G	(29)	7,6	—	44,9	1,1	—	38,0
Organic Psychosis							
T	(19)	12,5	23,1	6,2	5,2	4,4	1,3
G	(15)	3,1	—	71,1	0,7	—	87,0
Schizophrenia and Paranoid Psychosis							
T	(42)	30,0	14,8	7,7	17,4	9,7	3,9
G	(6)	2,8	—	27,0	2,3	—	66,0

need for admission and medication. In case of intolerably deviant behavior involuntary admission is still possible, although extremely rare.

To the Dutch observer, the most striking feature of mental health care in Trieste is the indivisible responsibility of one of the same mental health team for both inpatient, day, and outpatient care for all mentally ill people from their catchment area. The mental health center provides both first aid and long-term shelter. The staff, unlike in the Netherlands, cannot pass difficult patients on to other echelons of care. This requires great flexibility on the part of the staff.

Another feature is the lack of sharp boundaries between inpatient, day, and outpatient care. There are no fixed treatment programs to which the patient has to adapt. Care is adapted to the needs of the patient, which to the Dutch observer gives an impression of chaos, but it implies flexibility and continuity of care. In the Netherlands patients have fixed appointments, outside of which they easily become an embarrassment to the service, except in case of an emergency. Because of all this, acute and chronic patients do not occupy separate compartments of care; and growth or reduction of one compartment is immediately obvious to the staff because they are also responsible for all other compartments.

Finally, there is the way in which particularly young patients learn to define themselves, not as patients and as sick people, but as people temporarily in need of assistance.

In the Netherlands treatment programs have a strong identity to which the patient has to conform, for which he has to be motivated. The various components of the services are prominent as separate power blocks. For example, in recent times the intramural services (the mental hospitals) were perceived as too powerful. For this reason a counterbalance was sought by strengthening the social psychiatric services to the detriment of the mental hospital. The result of this is a battle for patients which has very little to do with their needs. Therefore, in Holland, compared with the situation in Trieste, the needs of services are too strong a factor in mental health care!

INDEX